EMS
THE JOB OF YOUR LIFE

DEVIN KERINS

EMS
THE JOB OF YOUR LIFE

DEVIN KERINS

VIVISPHERE
PUBLISHING

ISBN-10: 1-58776-122-X
ISBN-13: 978-1-58776-122-5

Library of Congress catalog number: 2002104135
Printed in the United States of America

VIVISPHERE PUBLISHING
A division of NetPub Corporation
675 Dutchess Turnpike, Poughkeepsie, NY 12603
www.vivisphere.com   (800) 724-1100

In Memory .... *ix*
Introduction .... *xv*

THE SHIFT BEGINS 1
THE EMS WORKER 5
RULES OF THE RIG 8
URBAN DIAGNOSIS 11
EMS HE SAID/SHE SAID 13
ABUSING MY KINDNESS 17
EMS Q & A 20
RANDOM THOUGHTS 23
GREAT RADIO MOMENTS 40
WORKING CODE 54
FUN WITH DOAs AND ODs 57
NURSING HOME NIGHTMARES 71
THE MATERNITY CALL 84
OB/GYN DISASTERS AND OTHER GENITAL ODDITIES 87
SEX INJURIES 97
RESPIRATORY DISTRESS 111
PSYCHIATRIC EMERGENCIES 114
CELLITUS 148
ASSAULTS 150
PERFECT END TO A PERFECT DAY? 163
MOTOR VEHICLE MISHAPS 165
DON'T GET MAD, GET EVEN 177
EMBARRASSING MOMENTS AND OTHER ASSORTED TALES 186
SIGNS YOU KNOW YOU'RE A WHACKER 202
ON THE MATTER OF STRESS 206
THAT'S A WRAP! 215
EMS TERMS AND ABBREVIATIONS 218

For my mother:
Forever in my heart, because of you, I am.

IN MEMORY

I usually love to put on the dress uniform of my department—the proud gray overcoat, the cap, the white gloves. I feel important; the uniform commands a certain respect especially when I'm marching side by side with my EMS brothers and sisters in a parade celebration.

Today we are marching past lines of knowing motorists who hang their heads or make signs of the cross and confused children who expect the fire trucks to blast their horns or smiling firefighters to wave back at them.

My EMS brother didn't die of a heart attack or in an automobile accident, but doing his job: trying to save lives. When all hell broke loose at the World Trade Center, and thousands upon thousands rushed out of the buildings, he ran in without hesitation.

When I found out he was among the missing, my jaw hit the floor. I wanted to break down and cry, but I knew I had to move on and continue to help the others in need. That's the job of an EMT.

As I stand here among my fellow coworkers, I want to cry again. Then I look behind me. For as far as I can see there are EMTs, firefighters, and police officers lined up in uniform. Many of them never knew him, never met him, never saw him work, or heard him laugh. They're here out of respect from the city, the suburbs and from towns I've never heard of. Normally, when one of us dies in the line of duty, the funeral procession could reach a mile long. However, too many of our brothers and sisters died in the line of duty this time, so many funerals being held that mourners cannot make them all. This is my third. I had to miss three others.

A part of EMT tradition is hoping for "The Big One"— that world-shaking disaster that would get our names and pictures in the paper; something to brag about later in our everyday runs.

On that fateful Tuesday morning in September, The Big One hit and nobody's bragging. Many of us will quit, others will have nightmares, and some may never be able to work again.

It's the desire to be a part of history and legend that drives people to The Big One. Nothing is more frustrating than being capable of helping and not being able to do anything. I'll remember seeing firefighters and EMTs from all over the country, as well as from France, at Ground Zero. Even though many of those helping weren't there when everything actually happened, everyone wanted to be a part of it. Even if I couldn't be there when it happened, I want to be able to say that I at least tried to do something.

That is why so many people from all over the state are attending this funeral. In some small way, by being here to honor my fallen brother and pay their respects, they are lending a hand. We feel a little better when we see the large procession. We know he's not forgotten.

It's also a reunion of sorts, a "who's who" of people who used to work at the department. Some left on good terms, others did not. This afternoon all differences are put aside to mourn the loss of a friend.

The Pipe and Drum Team from the fire and police departments leads the way. He wasn't Irish, but there's an old emergency services' saying: "We're all Irish at our funerals." The bagpipes and drums have been part of the tradition forever, it seems. I usually break down at the sound of bagpipes at a funeral. Not this time. My friend died a hero, doing his job, what I hope I would have done had I been in his shoes.

I think of his ailing mother he was taking care of and the fiancee he left behind and all who are saddened by this day. I pray they can take comfort: he died a hero.

I try to be strong. I know it's okay to cry. All around me I see men and women wiping tears from their eyes. It breaks my heart to see these strong people I work with every day breaking down. I know what's on their minds because I feel the same way: it could have been any one of us. Many, like me, are trying to fight back the tears. I know that when we go home and we're alone, the reality of what has happened will set it. The nightmares will come, the panic will set in, and the loneliness will overtake us.

I try to search for something to say, some magical words that might help take all the pain away. I think of the words the priest said to me when my mother passed way: "We must not be saddened because Patricia is no longer with us, for she is still, indeed, very much with us. We must get used to her being with us in a way we are not accustomed to." I remember being confused by this statement until we went to bury Mom. Everyone placed a rose on her coffin and a wind picked up and blew away all but the first seven roses—those from my father, my three brothers, my brother's fiancee, my mother's closest sister, and me. I'm not a very spiritual person, but this was a sign—as if she were telling us she is still here. I pray that my fallen brother's family and friends may see that he too is still with us, just in a different way now. When they close their eyes to sleep at night, perhaps they'll dream of him. Maybe they'll see a part of him in a newborn family member, or in themselves. Almost as much as my mother, he's a part of me and I'll never forget him.

The sun is shining, the wind gently blowing, and not a cloud is in the sky—not at all like how we feel. A James Taylor song plays over and over in my head.

'The sun shines on the funeral, the same as on a birth
The way it shines on everything that happens here on earth'

Outside the church there are floral arrangements. One with a New York Yankees' emblem is displayed next to one of a Dallas Cowboys helmet, his two favorite teams. There is a floral arrangement of our department patch, as well as the other department he worked for. The hearse pulls up, and we all stand respectfully and salute as the coffin is brought out, draped in an American flag.

We follow the family into the church and pack ourselves in. Every seat is taken and the standing room is filled. All along the walls and in the back rows are men and women in uniforms sobbing.

The mass begins. The priest says that my friend died while living. Truly living. So many of us go through life making plans for the future, but once in a while some of us may be faced with a situation where a future is uncertain and we must act without thinking of the consequences and just do what we have been taught to do. So many that day were forced to live. I wonder if I have ever really "lived." I recall some of the most dangerous moments I have faced on the job and wonder if any of them would be considered "living."

The priest goes on to quote from the Bible. There is no greater love than to give one's life for another. That's what he did. After pulling out two of his brothers, he could have rested and saved himself. Instead, he charged back in and the building collapsed.

After we receive communion, a lone bagpiper plays Amazing Grace and the sobbing starts again. I can't hold back anymore and I begin to weep. No longer will I be able to hear him on the radio, or shake his hand or laugh at him smoking a Cuban cigar while riding on duty with our Bike Team.

A respectful silence as his sister and best friend come forward to say some words. From an early age our EMT brother knew what he wanted to be. Joining a local first aid squad at age eleven, he became an explorer and began to learn about emergency medicine. He became an EMT at sixteen and a paramedic when he was twenty, and was named our supervisor at twenty-five.

The Commissioner of the New York State Department of Corrections reads a letter from New York City Mayor Rudy Giuliani, extending his deepest condolences to the family and friends and apologizing for not being able to attend.

Outside we line up again. Rows of paramedics, EMTs, firefighters, and police officers extend four or five deep and take up two city blocks. One of our administrators connects our EMS radio to the PA system on our ambulance. When the coffin is brought out, a dispatcher presses the alert tone and calls for my friend over the radio as if he were still alive and working. Then he announces, "Two-Fifty is out of service. May he rest in peace." If there had been a dry eye among us, there wasn't any more.

Today we mourn. Tomorrow we will be expected to be different. I fear the people of our city will not care about or be as moved by our loss as we are. Today we are considered heroes. People stop us on the street to thank us for what we did. We get free food delivered to our stations. People drop off extra football tickets for us. Women hit on us on calls. But for how long?

Life goes on. That's EMS, a demanding job for customers who accept no excuses for lateness or failure. A job that puts our lives on the line one way or another nearly every time we come to work. Are we expected to be emotionless robots when we set foot in that ambulance? That's not me or any other EMT, but sometimes, it seems, our customers want nothing else.

After the funeral we gather as all people do after funerals, to exchange condolences and hugs. We cry together, we mourn. But eventually, as all funerals do, the conversation goes back to the good times we had with the deceased. I remember how he made me try out for the Bike EMS team in my regular uniform pants. And then he laughed when my pants leg got caught in the cranks and I fell off the bike and rolled down the hill. And how he rode me the rest of the day because I had no change of uniform and had to work in my torn pants rife with grass stains. I remembered, too, how he smoothed things over with a patient's family when they accused me of being a racist just because I couldn't speak Spanish, and then busted my chops about it for a whole month.

Tomorrow we go back to work, enduring a loss that will not heal anytime soon. We must appear to carry on as if nothing had happened, to act professionally, and to care for our patients because that's EMS. That was his job, and no one did it better.

People often ask me "why?" Why do we put ourselves through these emotional roller coasters? Why do we continue to go into work everyday, with the knowledge that we may be called upon to make the ultimate sacrifice? Why do we, ordinary people, place ourselves in extraordinary situations? Because we love our jobs, and we love the people we work with. Every day has its own new adventures. As Dave Matthews sang:

> 'The space between the tears we cry
> Is the laughter that keeps us coming back for more.'

Tomorrow I return to work, and my EMS adventures will begin anew. I wouldn't have it any other way.

INTRODUCTION

If you're like me, you'll probably skip the intro and head right for the good stuff. But for those who like to read the book cover to cover, I'll try to be brief and entertaining.

I don't claim to be an expert in my field. I'm just a guy who loves what he does and has some stories to tell. As you have probably guessed from the title, I drive ambulances. I've been an Emergency Medical Technician (EMT) in New Jersey for over six years, and I have loved every minute of it.

Okay, so that might be stretching it a little. Let's just say I have never regretted my decision to become one. I would consider my attitude toward my job more of a love/hate relationship. But I'm getting ahead of myself.

I was born the third of four boys. We moved from Philadelphia to London, England, just after I was born. When I was seven, we moved back to the United States and lived in New Jersey. Because I was shy to begin with, and because I had a funny accent, the other kids teased me unmercifully. I became very introverted and spent most of my time reading, studying, and watching TV. On the upside to that, I was able to get good grades, I had good study habits, and eventually won a scholarship to college. On the downside, I became a world champion couch potato. Not only do I have a Bachelor's Degree and am working on a Master's, but I also have the uncanny and sometimes annoying ability to link everything that happens in my day to episodes of *The Simpsons* or *Married With Children*.

Growing up, I wanted to be many things, but being an EMT and saving lives was never one of them. I wanted to be a rock star, but the lack of any real musical talent ended that dream fast. I wanted to be a football star, but I have no real athletic ability outside of volleyball or video sports games. I even went to school to be a doctor. However, when I couldn't break double digits on my chemistry tests, I figured it was time to seek out another career.

One day, when I was a sophomore in high school, my older brother Sean and I were going to Burger King for lunch. He had been an EMT since his stint with the Merchant Marines. As we drove home, we happened upon an accident. Sean jumped out and helped the driver, a nun who had wrapped her car around a utility pole, out of the vehicle to safety. As I sat there in his car, eating my lunch *and his*, I thought, Hey, this is cool. I want to do that! So when I turned 16, I took the EMT class and the rest is history. Well, sort of.

I jumped right into Emergency Medical Services (EMS). I loved the rescue aspect of it. I'm always trying to challenge myself, so rescue work provides a great opportunity—both mentally and physically. I began taking courses in excavation trench collapse, building collapse, confined space rescue, rappelling, and vehicle extrication. Being a bit of a bookworm, I loved the idea that I had to take more classes every three years to keep my certification. There's always something interesting to take, like classes on drug awareness, mass casualty incidents, hazardous materials, and responding to terrorist attacks.

I love helping people, and that's what I think this job is all about. Some may say the job is all about saving lives, but we don't always do that. It's not that frequently that I get to actually snatch someone back from the greedy clutches of death. When that does happen though, it's the best feeling in the world.

But it can also be rewarding by being the calming influence on the family and ensuring the patient gets to the hospital safely or teaching people how to help themselves if the situation arises again. Most of all, it's helping someone by being the person who can convince the patient that everything *will* be okay.

I love this job because I know that I am making a difference, no matter how small, in someone's life. But most of all, I must admit, because I get to drive fast and obnoxiously. Plus . . . chicks dig the uniform!

So why do I sometimes hate my job? There are a few things that get me upset: the pay, the long hours, being unappreciated, and the feeling of being a glorified taxi.

The one thing I have noticed about *all* people working in emergency services is that they love to tell stories. Every one of us has experienced some things that we are dying to tell people. And the most common reaction from the people we tell is utter disbelief. That makes the story telling even better.

I have a few hopes with this book. The first hope I have is that people who are in the emergency services field—be they EMTs, police officers, firefighters, etc.—will read this and relate to it. I want them to know that they are not alone in their experiences. *Absurd things happen to all of us!* The second hope is that people who have family or friends in the emergency services field will read this and wonder what their loved ones have seen. We all have stories, and we're all dying to tell them. My third hope is that people who have no connection to the emergency services field will become interested enough to find out more. My final hope is that this will be a major best seller, making me millions, and allowing me to retire on a tropical island at an early age. Okay, so that might be farfetched. I'll just settle for the first three.

A word of advice before you begin: To help the reader who might not be familiar with the way EMTs talk, I have tried to write this in such a way that you may be able to understand it. I have included a glossary of terms in the back, both serious and humorous, to help you understand the book. Please read that first.

Here's my disclaimer for the entire book: In this book I think I mock everyone possible, including myself. The thoughts and opinions expressed in these pages are my own and even some that are not my own that I made up for a laugh. They do not reflect the opinions of the organizations or those of the members of the organizations with which I am affiliated. The names and locations of these events have been changed to protect the innocent, as well as the guilty. I do not condone some of the actions that are described in this book; I just get a kick out of hearing and retelling them. This book is in no way an attack on any group of people, but it does poke fun at some of the stereotypes that EMS workers put on their patients.

I believe that I am a product of my environment. Having grown up with three brothers and working in an urban environment, my language tends to slip and I cuss like a sailor.

To my knowledge, all of the stories in this book are true. This book is solely meant in fun. And finally, I swear on a stack of Bibles that no animals were hurt during the making of this book . . . well, except for those two rabid dogs and a runaway deer—but they had it coming!

Some of this may shock you, some of it may disturb you, and, hopefully, some of it will make you laugh. Just remember that I didn't really write this book; my patients did. I just put it on paper.

THE SHIFT BEGINS

It's 4:30 in the morning. The alarm clock wakes me out of an incredible dream. One moment, I'm relaxing on a sun-filled beach, ten yards from the breaking waves, sipping on fruity alcohol–filled drinks when suddenly a horrible buzzing snaps me back into reality.

My back cracks as I sit up in bed. I do a little twist to get all the kinks out. I breathe a sigh of relief as I feel my spine pop back into place. Years of lifting heavy patients have wreaked havoc on my faithful backbone. I fumble for the glass of water I left next to the bed and try to swish out the taste of morning breath. Sleep crust gets removed from my eyes and it's time to hit the shower. The cloudiness in my head reminds me that I didn't get nearly enough sleep last night. *What else is new?*

The cold water wakes me up. Unfortunately, I didn't want it to be cold, and I take the lack of warm water as a harbinger of things to come. I bury my face in my hands. That's a position not at all uncommon to the EMS worker. *Please let it be a good day!*

After the shower, I search desperately for a pair of matching socks. *Where do they all go anyway? Is there a mysterious singles' club for socks? I know all the missing socks are getting together somewhere in my house and laughing at me.* Looking at the time, I grab the first two socks that look remotely alike.

One final glance in the mirror. *Got your watch?* Check. *Your stethoscope?* There it is. *Hair looks good?* Not too shabby. *Uniform neatly ironed?* Hell no, but close enough. *Boots polished?* Absolutely not. I spend so much time in those things that they won't stay polished more than an hour anyway. Why bother?

I pull into the station to find my ambulance where I left it. As usual, the night guys have plundered my truck. *Dirty pirates.* I curse and yell as if they were there. Then I throw a box of latex gloves across the back. That makes me feel a little better; wanton destruction usually does. Now it's time to make a list of what they did leave me.

Lucky for me, they left the not-so-important equipment, such as sterile water, tape, and hydrogen peroxide. All the really important stuff, like the oxygen masks and bandages, have been removed from my vehicle. I also make a note to get more emesis basins in case any of my patients decide to blow chunks.

I make up the stretcher. Next I check my defibrillator. The self-test mode on the machine tells me everything is working fine. *That's nice, hope I don't have to find out.*

Inside is taken care of; now it's time for the outside. First I check to make sure the lifting devices are there. Both are fine. Next I check the backboards. Not surprisingly, there are no backboards. *Got to have those.* I see another ambulance that no one is using and decide to grab the boards off of that. *Hey, what goes around comes around!*

My partner shows up. We dispense with the usual pleasantries of "Hey, how was your evening? That's great, mine sucked," and it's off to tackle another day of making a difference.

I call on the radio to my dispatcher and tell him I'm in service. My stomach grumbles. *Wish I had time to eat breakfast this morning.* He cheerily greets me with a friendly hello and my first assignment of the day. On the outside of 123 Main Street, there's a man lying in the bushes, possibly not moving.

I just got in, and already I'm working. This is not a good sign!

At 6:30 in the morning, there aren't too many cars on the road. However, I know that the number of cars on the road means absolutely nothing in terms of how bad my response will be.

I pull out of the station and turn left. No one on the road yet. *That's good.* I hang a right at the first stoplight. A driver up ahead sees me coming and gently guides his car over to the right side of the road. I glide effortlessly past him down the hill. I swing a left onto a side street. What I see enrages me.

Someone has double-parked his car in the street. The driver is still in it, with the seat reclined. Next to him, on his left, is a space wide enough to find his car and mine easily. *Would it have been too much trouble for you to have parallel parked?* I wail on the siren. He wakes up, groggily starts the car, and drives up the street. He pulls over into a very small spot, yet he is still blocking the road. I hit the siren again, and he moves. I manage to pass him, and he flips me the middle finger. *Gee sir, I'm sorry I inconvenienced you.*

I make it onto Main Street without any further problems. I take the spotlight out of its holder and try to shine it along the ground to look for my patient. Not surprisingly, the spotlight doesn't work. *Nothing works when you really want it to.*

I see my patient lying in a bunch of thick bushes. I get out and approach cautiously. The torn leather jacket, faded jeans, and stench of sweat and stale whiskey tip me off right away. It's Mikey Jones, one of my regulars. I know he's a mean drunk, so I give him a little tap with my foot. Not a kick, just a nudge to wake him up. He stirs, and I step back a little. He gets up and stands in front of me dazed for a moment. As he opens his mouth to speak, a couple of leaves fall out of his mouth and catch on his red beard. He starts to stagger towards me. He stumbles and I reach out to catch him. He falls into my arms and, without making a sound, throws up all over me.

All this fun and it's only 6:40. Eleven hours and twenty minutes left. Maybe I should have stayed in bed. I shrug that thought off.

This is my job. Welcome to it.

THE EMS WORKER

What drives someone to become an Emergency Medical Technician or Paramedic? What sane, rational person would ever want to work in a job that involves long hours, poor pay, and dealing with death and disease? No sane person, that's who!

I firmly believe that every one of us in this business is a little screwy. And in some cases, such as yours truly, extremely screwy.

Job Description:

Care for the sick and injured. This involves dealing with death and other stressful situations. One must be willing to go long periods without sleep, food, or potty breaks. Be expected to race madly across town in all forms of weather at all hours of the day for a variety of calls. Be in decent shape to climb endless numbers of stairs with heavy equipment, then come back down those stairs with all the equipment and a patient. This can be avoided, however, if one is adept at delegating orders and shirking responsibilities.

Benefits:

The benefits package is subject to the area in which one works. Some may get full medical/dental coverage, 401Ks, and IRAs. The really lucky ones will get discounts from the clerks at the local coffee shops and convenience stores.

Pay Scale:

A predictable pattern: Start off with nothing, end up with nothing. Don't be surprised to hear uncontrollable weeping coming from fellow employees when picking up a paycheck. Also, it is not at all uncommon to hear actual laughter coming from the paycheck itself.

Stomach:

One must be able to withstand a barrage of the foulest stenches, goriest scenes, and a wide range of greasy fast foods and bad coffee. Or nothing at all for too long.

Bladder:

Must be able to hold tight for hours and be able to empty immediately as soon as there is a break in the calls. It must also be strong and not let loose because of the way one's partner drives.

Sleeping patterns:

Endure long periods without plus the ability to fall asleep anywhere. Not narcolepsy, just being able to doze off when there is a pause in the calls.

Verbal skills:

Patients will expect you to speak whatever language they do. If one can speak foreign languages, that's excellent. But one of the most important phrases in EMS is "Who here speaks English?"

Attitude:

Be able to adapt to your partner. There is nothing worse than being stuck with someone you can't stand for eight or twelve hours. Be sensitive to the needs of the patient and the patient's family and remain professional at all times. This is especially true when dealing with extremely stressful situations, such as when a patient calls the ambulance because he has an ingrown toe nail. Be able to laugh off the angry comments made by the patient or bystanders.

Reflexes:

The ability to dodge a variety of flying objects, including but not limited to: insults, bullets, vomit, punches, and human waste products.

But, above all else, the individual must be able to laugh at absurdity. It's a roller coaster ride with ups and downs, moments when you want to laugh and moments when you want to scream, times when you want to get off and times when you never want to leave. But through it all, it is possible to enjoy this job. In fact, it *can* be enjoyable sometimes. Sometimes . . .

RULES OF THE RIG

There are certain unwritten rules that must be adhered to at all times on the ambulance. I feel compelled to write these down and codify them. If I could have my way, I would post them on the truck for both patients and partners to see. Breaking any of these cardinal rules is subject to swift and severe punishment.

Patient Rules:

1. Thou shalt not blow chunks in my ambulance. You may throw up on yourself, on your friends, on your furniture, or into some type of approved container, but at no time is vomit to touch the floor of my truck.
2. Thou shalt not whine unless given expressed permission from me to do so.
3. You called me, therefore you have no right to complain about my driving!
4. I don't care if your taxes or insurance pay my salary, you're in my world now!
5. Do not ask me stupid questions. I do not know how long you will be at the hospital; I do not know if your

leg is broken; I do not get paid a lot to do this; and yes, I have seen dead bodies—grotesque bodies in all stages of decomposition. I think that covers the answers to most of the questions.

6. Everyone walks to the truck unless they have a very good reason to be carried.

7. I don't care whose fault the accident or fight was. Do not bore me with these details unless I ask for them.

8. You may not bring carry-on luggage with you. I am not a taxi. If you had the time and energy to pack those bags, I doubt if you really needed an emergency ambulance.

9. Just because I drive you to the hospital does not mean that you will be seen any faster. If I hear you say those words to me, I will do everything in my power to make sure you spend as much time as possible in the waiting room.

10. I cannot accept tips for my services. However, if some money should happen to fall on the floor . . .

Partner Rules:

1. No whining unless given expressed permission to do so.

2. The driver is the sole controller of which radio stations the crew listens to. The driver may give up this right, but the other crew members may not touch the radio until he does so.

3. The new guy will do all the running up and down the stairs for equipment.

4. When two men are working together, it is the responsibility of both crew members to alert the other when they see attractive females.

5. When you pass gas in the truck, you must apologize for it immediately or blame the patient if you have one. Responsibility must be assigned and windows must be opened quickly.

6. The other crew members are not allowed to complain about the driving. If you think you can do better, by all means go ahead.
7. Since the driver has to make all the decisions about where to go and what to listen to, the crew chief is responsible for deciding where to eat. "I don't know" is not an acceptable answer.
8. Thou shalt not volunteer to take a call for another unit unless the call is on the outside or on the first floor of a building.
9. Thou shalt expect and graciously welcome any teasing you receive for stupid things you happen to do.
10. Everyone walks unless they can prove otherwise.

URBAN DIAGNOSIS

These are some of the better slaughterings of the English language I have come across in the field. (Or maybe when people have emergencies to deal with, they can't talk straight.)

Am'lance: the vehicle an EMT drivers, a.k.a. **Bamb'lance.**

She's Bacardi arrested: She's in cardiac arrest.

He's carjack arrested: He's in cardiac arrest.

I take Dilut'ns: I take the seizure medication Dilantin.

He fell out: We believe this is to have a seizure, but it is also used to say that someone has passed out.

He's got the Hi Five: He's HIV positive.

I gots the High Blood: I have high blood pressure.

He's on the Lexus: He takes the high blood pressure medication Lasix.

Mr. Am'lance Man: The crew of the ambulance.

She's got the Package: She has AIDS.

I have a problem in my Pantry: I'm having pain in my pancreas. (And yes, I did think for a minute that she actually had something wrong with the closet in her kitchen.)

I take Peanut Butter Balls: I take the seizure medication Phenobarbital.

He's got Scissors: He has seizures.

She's got the Shakes: She has seizures.

I got the Sugars: I have Diabetes.

I think I'm allergic to the Water Chicken: I believe I am allergic to duck.

I have fire balls shooting out of my eucharist: I still have no idea what this one is. I think it is fibral cysts of the uterus.

EMS HE SAID/SHE SAID

This chapter hopes to help the reader understand what the patient, EMT, or paramedic means when he or she says certain things.

The patient says: This is kind of embarrassing.
The patient means: This is REALLY embarrassing.

The patient says: No, I don't have any medical problems.
The patient means: That is to say I have no medical problems I wish to tell you about. I am actually HIV positive, have gonorrhea, and have this unidentifiable rash on my genitals.

The patient says: No, I don't take any medicine.
The patient means: I take enough medicine to stop a charging rhino, but since I can't remember them, I'm not telling you.

The patient says: I don't know how this happened.
The patient means: I was doing something I know I shouldn't have been doing, so I'll just play dumb.

The patient says: I don't want to talk about it.
The patient means: I've done something *really* dumb and I am too ashamed to talk about it.

The patient says: I don't know how much I've had to drink tonight.
The patient means: I stopped counting after the third 40 oz. malt liquor.

The patient says: I want to go to detox.
The patient means: I'm cold, I'm hungry, I need a shower, and I know the hospital will provide me with one. Don't fool yourself into thinking I might actually stop drinking.

The patient says: I weight about . . .
The patient means: I am lying to you. I weight at least twenty pounds more than what I am telling.

The patient says: I can't walk.
The patient means: I probably could walk, but I don't want to.

The patient says: Do you want to see?
The patient means: I have these festering boils on my ass and I want to ruin your dinner by showing them to you.

The patient says: I don't want to go to XYZ hospital. They don't do anything for me when I go there.
The patient means: (A) I'm still in shock that they didn't think my toothache was an emergency last time. (B) They never give me anything good to take when I go there.

The patient says: It's been bothering me for a week, but it just got worse tonight.
The patient means: My medical insurance won't pay for

this if I don't come in by ambulance. Since there is nothing good on TV tonight, and I knew you were napping, I figured now would be the best time to call.

The patient says: You need to give me exactly 1.5 mg of Demerol.
The patient means: I am a junkie.

The EMT says: How much did you drink tonight?
The EMT means: No matter how much you say you had to drink tonight I will not believe you, you lush!

The EMT says: Just to let you know, if you are coming with us, you're going to be waiting awhile.
The EMT means: This is absolute BS and I don't feel like wasting my time taking you over there.

The EMT says: Can you walk?
The EMT means: I really don't think I could carry you without dropping a testicle.

The EMT says: XYZ hospital is much better for this problem and you might not be waiting there that long.
The EMT means: That hospital (A) is closer to where my dinner is waiting for me, (B) is closer to the station and I get off in twenty minutes, or (C) has a much cleaner bathroom and I have to pee so bad my back teeth are floating.

The EMT says: His blood pressure was unobtainable.
The EMT means: I didn't feel like looking.

The EMT says: I couldn't hear what his lungs sounded like.
The EMT means: My stethoscope was in the truck.

The EMT says: I'll take your word for it.
The EMT means: That was the most disgusting thing anyone has ever described to me. No, I do not want to see that!

When the paramedic says to the EMT: Do you need us?
The paramedic means: I don't feel like doing any work so please cancel me.

The EMT says: And what do the voices in your head tell you?
The EMT means: I'm bored and I need a good laugh.

The EMT says: No, I don't think you're crazy.
The EMT means: Yeah, actually I think you're *really* crazy

The EMT says: You weight 250 lbs., okay.
The EMT means: 250 lbs., my ass, which leg?

The EMT says: No, no, don't be embarrassed.
The EMT means: Be embarrassed, be very embarrassed. In fact, I'm going to tell all my friends about your misfortune and we'll all have a good laugh. Come to think of it, I'll use it in a book and make millions off of your distress.

ABUSING MY KINDNESS

The day has barely begun and I've already gone through one uniform. *And people wonder why how I can be so cynical about my job.* The uniform has now been changed and I'm in search of something to eat. That doesn't last too long, though. *Now I'm regretting not packing some snacks before I left the house.*

We are dispatched for a man not feeling well. He lives on the second floor of an apartment building that is starting to slip into disrepair. The elevator is poorly lit; one of the fluorescent bulbs has burnt out. There is a thin layer of fresh urine on the red elevator floor. An empty vodka bottle is broken in the corner. I hold my breath as the elevator ever-so-slowly moves up one floor. *Sometimes it pays to take the stairs.*

The door of the apartment is unlocked and we let ourselves in. The patient is lying on the bed. He is complaining that he has been throwing up and having diarrhea for the past few days. He says he can't walk. My usual response is, "If you can't walk, then how did you make it to the bathroom? Did you go on yourself?" One whiff of the patient tells me that there's no need to use that line.

We assess the patient, get all of his vital information, and sit him up in the stair chair. "Sir, do you have everything?" I ask.

"Can you get my keys? They are on the table."

"Sure, no problem." I find the keys and hand them to him.

"Can you just make sure my windows are closed?"

"Okay, hold on." I quickly look around the apartment and make sure the windows are closed. "Okay, sir, they're closed. Are you ready now?"

"You didn't check all of them."

"Yes I did."

"No. Make sure they are all closed."

"But sir . . ."

"No buts!" He reaches out and grabs hold of the doorway. "I'm not going until you check them again."

Seeing that I am about to snap, my partner intervenes and checks the windows. "See, I told you I closed them." I say. "Are you ready to go now?"

"Yes. Thank you."

We begin to wheel him out of the house. He suddenly reaches out again.

"Wait!" His cry startles me and I fumble and let go of the chair. It snaps forward. "Ouch, you idiot! Do you have any idea what you are doing?" He yells at me.

"What the hell were you yelling at?"

"My cat."

"What about your cat?"

"Make sure I fed him."

"No, no, no! That's it, we're leaving."

"Hey, easy. You guys are supposed to be public servants. This is not what I call serving the public."

"Look, you miserable . . ." I start to yell at him, but my partner cuts me off.

"Sir, we have to get going. You won't be gone long enough for the cat to starve."

"Fine," he acquiesces, "but you guys should change your attitudes. Anytime someone wants me to do something for them, I do it. No questions asked."

Oh really? Then again, you've got no clue what I feel like asking you to do right now!

EMS Q & A

Here are some of the more commonly asked questions that EMTs are asked, as well as what I think everyone's answer should be. After hearing these questions so many times, you just want to be a wise ass.

Q: Will you hold this for me?
A: No, I will not hold that bucket of puke for you. You produced it, now enjoy it!

Q: You have to do what I say. Don't you know my taxes pay your salary?
A: Choose which is appropriate for you:
(1) No, you're taxes don't pay my salary; I'm a volunteer.
(2) No, you're taxes don't pay my salary; I work for the hospital. Your medical insurance pays my salary. Oh, what's that? You have no insurance? Then shut up!
(3) Thank you for reminding me of that. However, while I don't doubt that you pay taxes, your taxes don't pay my salary; they merely contribute to it. If you paid my salary, you would be paying well over

$26,000 in taxes a year. If that were true, I suggest you move.

(4) I pay taxes, too. Which means I pay my own salary. Which means I do what *I* want.

Q: Have you ever seen a dead body?
A: Sure I have! Who do you think was lying on that stretcher just before you?

Q: Can you just check my blood pressure?
A: You mean to tell me you made me race all the way across town to check your blood pressure?

Q: Is my blood pressure okay?
A: That depends: is it always *that* high?

Q: Is it broken?
A: How the hell should I know? I left my X-ray goggles in the other ambulance.

Q: You think I'm crazy, don't you?
A: Yeah, pretty much.

Q: I can't walk; can you carry me?
A: Let me see, ma'am. You're six-five and 350 pounds, and you called because you have had a cold for the past two weeks. No f—ing way will I carry you!
            or
A: So answer me this: you've been lying on that couch for the past ten hours, and now you expect me to carry you? Do you have a toilet attached to that couch? How is it possible you can make it upstairs to the bathroom, but not ten feet out to the ambulance?

Q: Did you need to see this?

A: Well, it would have been nice to see that *Do Not Resuscitate* order fifteen minutes ago, before we went against *all* of his wishes.

Q: Do you have to go to school for this?
A: No, not at all. This stuff just comes natural to everyone.

Q: You do know what you are doing, right?
A: Yeah, sure. I mean, heck, the first five times I failed the test were just warm-ups.

Q: Do I need to go to the hospital?
A: If you have to ask whether you need to, I guess the answer would be no.

Q: Do you get paid a lot of money?
A: Yeah, right. In fact I'm moving into my summerhouse in the Hamptons next week.

Q: Is he okay?
A: Well, your baby swallowed a quarter and he doesn't seem to be having any trouble breathing. So, yeah, I think he'll be okay. It just needs to pass through his system. Now, if he shits two dimes and a nickel, then be worried.

RANDOM THOUGHTS

The following are random thoughts on the matter of EMS. A lot of it was taken from actual conversations with other EMTs. Most of it comes from what I thought up in my free time. (Gees, do I have no life?)

> DISCLAIMER: I am in no way making fun of any group directly, just the stereotypes.

The further away from ground level the patient is, the more likely it is that the patient will be of considerable weight. This does not hold true if the building has an elevator. So, if you have a patient on the fifth floor of a walk-up with no elevators, the greater the chance that the patient's leg weighs more than your whole body.

The first patient you are called for just after recovering from a back injury will weight at least 350 pounds.

Large patients will always find humor in the fact that you are about to collapse lifting them.

Doesn't anyone get sick on the first floor?

Patients who *can't* walk *will* try; patients who *can* walk *never* try.

Full moons *do* bring out the crazies.

When you are carrying a patient down the stairs and you are upset that he is heavy, take heart in the fact that it could be worse: you could be carrying him *up* the stairs! And if you are carrying a heavy patient up the stairs, don't worry, it could be worse: the patient could be going to bathroom on himself. And if you are carrying a heavy patient that is going to the bathroom on himself . . . Point is, it could always be worse.

The minute you concede to the fact that things could get worse, they DO get worse.

When you drop a piece of important equipment, it will always land in the most unreachable place.

If two pieces equipment look alike in storage but serve completely different purposes, i.e. the bag of splints and the Reeves, the rookie will grab the wrong one when you need it most.

Sick people don't bitch, but the one who has waited four weeks to call you for the back pain she has been having is the first to demand your supervisor's number so she can complain about how long it took you to get there.

Despite the pinpoint pupils and fresh needle tracks up the arm, your patient swears to have no idea what heroin is.

All EMS personnel are Jerry Springer Addicts.

Why is it that reality-based TV shows, like *Rescue 911*, never seem that realistic?

No matter how fast you get to someone's house, they never think it's fast enough.

Are there any medical groups that endorse beating common sense into patients who need it? If so, call me.

Something they won't teach you in EMT class: "Are you kidding me?" and "So, why did you wait until now to call?" are two of the most commonly asked assessment questions.

Having a baby, just like driving a car or wearing Spandex, should require a license.

What kind of a world do we live in when 13 year old girls are becoming pregnant? More disturbing, though, what kind of world do we live in when the men getting these girls pregnant are at least 23 years old? I'll admit I was no winner with the ladies when I was in high school, but never once did the thought of cruising the local kindergarten for dates cross my mind.

When given the choice of going to the hospital or going to jail, the prisoner will always choose the hospital. They just think they get off the hook if they spontaneously contract the plague.

Your call volume will increase noticeably the first weekend of each month. This coincides with the distribution of welfare checks. The calls will follow a logical pattern:
Friday night: Increased numbers of intoxicated persons, overdoses, and bar fights.
Saturday morning: This will be an incredibly quiet period for you, so much so that you may be lulled into a false sense of

security and believe that this will be a quiet day. But don't be fooled: come noon or one o'clock, they will all wake up hung over from the night before and create mayhem.

Saturday afternoon: This will be a period of increased domestic abuse.

Saturday night: More intoxicated people, overdoses, bar fights, and even a few drug-induced crazy people. There will also be a rise in suicide attempts.

Sunday morning: Now you begin to find younger DOAs, usually the result of a weekend's worth of partying.

How can I prove this theory? I can't, but I sound pretty smart saying it, right?

Never cut a Down Feather coat. You'll regret it if you do.

Seventy-five percent of all BLS patients are susceptible to the *EMT Mind Trick*. They will agree to go to any hospital you want them to go to, provided that you utter these words: "Well, last time I was in XYZ Hospital, there weren't too many people. That was only a half hour ago, so you probably won't be waiting that long."

If the elevator in a housing project that leads to the floor you want to go to (because they usually only go to odd floors or evens) is out of service, it is more likely that the one elevator will be flooded with urine.

Why is there always a gold-trimmed Lexus in the parking lot of a housing project? That means that you are either (A) a drug dealer, or (B) seriously in need of a priority re-evaluation. If you can afford to make those kinds of car payments, you can afford to live somewhere where there isn't feces in the stairwells.

The likelihood of a call coming increases greatly when

you (A) are just about to sit down and eat, (B) have 10 minutes left of your shift and something really important planned afterwards, or (C) you are debating whether or not you need to stop and use the bathroom.

The fact that my ambulance was built by the lowest bidder provides absolutely no comfort or confidence in the safety of the vehicle.

Whoever invented Haldol and Narcan should be made saints.

People with chest pains or numbness in the arms will often be in denial or afraid that they are having a heart attack or stroke. Therefore, these people usually don't call an ambulance for themselves. Also, when a patient is seriously injured, you usually have to fight tooth and nail to get a look at the injury site.
So why is it that a patient in no real emergency with nasty, unidentifiable bumps or rashes or some new and amazingly nauseating disease will be more than happy to expose you to it?

If you are homeless and living in a public facility, such as a subway station, that is open 24 hours a day, why can't you use the facility's bathroom instead of pissing on yourself?

Fashion sense is the first thing to go when you lose your mind.

It won't rain until you forget your jacket.

You won't get dirty if you have a spare uniform in the car. You will be covered in nasty person junk if you don't.

You will have some of the weirdest conversations with your partner, such as whether or not blind people have to pick up after their seeing-eye dogs or why that man is walking that pit bull with a baseball bat in the other hand.

Patients who know the system will often throw things in when calling that they think will make you come faster. For example: you get dispatched to the broken finger, with chest pains, or the person with a stubbed toe who is still actively seizing.

Parking your ambulance in a highly visible spot to get lunch or to people-watch seems to be an open invitation for the craziest or most annoying people to come and strike up a conversation with you.

Why do people stick their arms out the window to wave an ambulance past? I'm gonna pass you anyway. I'm just waiting for one of them to get an arm ripped off.

I'll never understand why people sit in their car in the middle of the street, not move, and cover their ears when you hit the sirens trying to pass them. I'll also never get those people who cover their ears and walk out in front of an ambulance. Pretending not to hear me is not going to change the fact that I am about to run you over.

The worst group of drivers on the road is not teenagers or the elderly; it's cab drivers. (Especially New York City cabbies!)

No matter what city or town you are in, the closer you get to the hospital, the worse the bumps in the street get. It also seems that the richer the area you are in, the deeper the potholes are.

A patient will deny having any medical problems when you ask them for a past medical history, but give you a list a mile long of medication when you ask what they are taking.

An interesting twist to this is the patient that lists every possible medical condition they have ever had, EX-CEPT for the really important things: "Well, let's see, I had back surgery when I was twelve, I have an in-grown toenail, I had a cold last year, my wisdom teeth removed twelve years ago . . ."

"But you have medicine for seizures."

"Oh, yeah, I have seizures too." (Right before they begin to convulse.)

Emergency services as we know them would grind to a screeching halt if Dunkin Donuts went out of business.

The people you see walking around the streets that "look" crazy usually are crazy and you'll be dispatched for them within the hour.

If you pass a frequent flyer walking down the street, or utter his name in conversation with your partner, you *will* pick him up two hours later.

A patient's "friend" or "cousin" who appears really con-cerned about the patient and yells at you for working too slowly will *not* know the patient's name.

Bystander Amnesia: Bystanders never know what hap-pened. Every single gangbanger on the block watched the shooting, stabbing, or beating, even cheered it on. But, no-body ever saw a thing.

People will never have a problem with their asthma un-til they run out of or lose their inhaler.

The Correlation of Weather to Call Location: When it is snowing or raining, the majority of your calls will be on the outside. When it is hot, the majority of your calls will be inside houses where the patient doesn't bathe and the air conditioner is broken.

The Rule of Doctors on Scene: The person on scene who identifies himself as a doctor is either a proctologist, an ophthalmologist, or something of absolutely no use to you.

Every bystander is a self-schooled traumatologist, and everyone on the scene thinks they know your job better than you do.

Family members of a patient with diabetes will think that every problem is directly related to his sugar level.
"He's having chest pains; it's probably his sugar!"—"He's bleeding from his rectum. Quick, someone check his sugar!"

There is a global conspiracy out there: People will step over the stranger's body laying in the hallway and wait until you are about to eat to call you. "He's been laying outside my door since I got home a couple of hours ago and I'm worried because he's not moving." So why didn't they call when they got home? *Because they know!*

Why do dispatchers tell you not to enter a scene if there is a violent and emotionally unstable patient present? Isn't that understood? Like I woke up this morning thinking, "Gee, today would be a great day to get my ass beat."

The cross street your dispatcher gives you for reference will always be four streets off. Or, the landmark they give you for reference no longer exists.

Dispatchers will always find a way to mispronounce even the most common street names.

When you can't understand if your dispatcher said Wright Street, Bright Street, or Light Street, you will always pick the wrong one.

For the knocking dispatchers get, I have to give them credit. Their job is certainly the hardest. There is no evidence if I happen to laugh in someone's face. Their phone lines, however, are taped. How they do it is beyond me. I could never be a dispatcher. I would get fired for saying something dumb, like "He's dead? Okay, I'll send someone. Call me back if anything changes."

If you are a dispatcher and someone calls saying he is in cardiac arrest, chances are *very* good that he isn't.

The family of the patient who lives three blocks from the hospital will wait for you to show up at the house, complain that they could have taken the patient to the hospital faster, then sign a refusal and drive themselves to the hospital.

Alright, someone explain this to me: You're eight to nine months pregnant. You start having abdominal pains. Then, magically, your water breaks. Doesn't that mean you are in labor? So why, then, do you drive yourself to the doctor's office only to call an ambulance from there instead of just driving yourself to the hospital?

If you were to take a poll of people who are deathly allergic to bee stings, you would probably find that ninety-five percent of them are carrying expired epinephrine kits, or none at all.

If neither you nor your partner speaks Spanish, the majority of your patients will only be able to speak Spanish.

Patients who only speak Spanish will be mortified that you don't.

If both you and your partner speak Spanish, then you will get patients that speak French, German, Ugandan, whatever.

Patients who may not have finished much formal schooling tend to use huge words to convey their thoughts in an effort to feel as smart as they think you are. The only problem is that these words are either (A) the wrong term for the situation but still close, or (B) totally and completely wrong or not even a word.

For example: I had an assault victim at a police station. He was beat up pretty good, and the police asked if he could identify his attackers. He said, "Yeah, I can tell you who did it, but you gotsta keep me monogamous."

"Monogamous?" the cop said. "I got nothing to do with that."

If the term is for something *really* important, the translation will come at the most inopportune time.

For example: I had a patient in respiratory distress. I asked his wife what medical problems he had. She said he had "toxicplastisenema." (That is, of course, the phonetic spelling because I doubt that's even a real word.) I asked her what that was, but she only decided to answer me right after he threw up all over me and went into cardiac arrest. "Oh yeah," she said. "Do you know what that is?" *Of course not, please enlighten me Mrs. Thesaurus.* "That's AIDS!"

Anyone who is taking more than five medications at one time is a miracle of modern science. Its a wonder that the five of them don't interact and kill the patient.

The idiot who wraps his own car around a telephone pole is the first person to complain about your driving to the hospital.

No matter how many calls you've been on, no matter how many miles you have driven at breakneck speeds in your ambulance without crashing, your mother or father will always complain about your driving the second they sit in your car.

The person who is illegally doubled parked will inevitably give you dirty looks and curse you out when you tell him to move.

The oldest, slowest person in the city will decide that *now* is a good time to cross the street just as you are barreling down the road.

The patient who calls you right before you are supposed to go home will (A) require significant ALS intervention that strands you on the scene for over a half an hour, or (B) take a half an hour to decide whether or not he wants to go to the hospital, then decide to go to the furthest possible hospital from your station.

People who buy vicious, blood thirsty animals as pets, i.e. a pitbull, then treat them like crap, barely feed them, and beat them, will be the most shocked that Rover just tried to devour their child.

If you call ahead to the hospital and tell them that your patient is actively seizing, by the time you get to the hospital, the patient will have stopped, making you look like a moron.

All calls for unconscious/unresponsive patients between

5 and 9 in the morning will always (A) be found in the bathroom, or (B) be DOA.

All emotionally disturbed persons (EDPs) who hear voices can be classified into four groups:
1. Those that hear voices that tell them to kill themselves or someone else
2. Those that hear voices that tell them to hurt themselves or others
3. Those that hear voices that tell them to start fires
4. Those that hear voices that tell them to take their clothes off and direct traffic.

Anyone who has worked in a city, in any capacity, has come across the four urban dialects.
1. **The We-bes:** These are the young hoodlums that hang out on the corner in the middle of the night. "We be doing nuttin officer!"
2. **The Do-Das or Do-Yas:** These are the annoying people who interrupt your ability to eat dinner. "Esscuse me, do da bus stop here?" or more annoying, "Do-yas have some change?"
3. **Mon-backs:** These interrupt your ability to sleep. Just when you get comfortable, you hear these guys yelling to the garbage truck or delivery truck, "Mon back! Mon back!" This goes on so long that you feel like the truck only goes in reverse.
4. **Geese:** Those people who, no matter what you ask them, they answer you by honking "Hhhuuhh?"

If you are at an accident scene on a Friday night and don't find someone drunk, look harder. You've obviously overlooked someone.

Why do people get into an accident, get out of the car

to walk around, smoke a cigarette, and yell at the other person, then get back *into* the car and then complain they can't move?

A single vehicle accident on a backwoods road will usually be the result of a patient dodging a small animal. Plus, if the patient was swerving to avoid hitting a small animal, they will usually be driving a sport utility vehicle or a boat on wheels.

I had a patient that wrapped his car around a concrete bridge abutment on a backwoods road near Princeton, New Jersey. He was driving a large Cadillac, you know, the kind your grandparents drive. He hit the bridge abutment so hard that the engine block was sitting in the passenger seat, and he had been ejected out the side of the car. But his luck didn't stop there. When he was forced out of the car, he fell 10 feet down the embankment.

Now, his car is totaled, he's in the ambulance waiting for the helicopter to be flown to a trauma center, and his excuse: "I saw the deer up by the bend in the road (about 50 feet ahead of where he hit the bridge) and I didn't want to hit it, so I swerved."

In Princeton, it is illegal to hunt deer. So the deer run rampant, like tall rats with antlers. I'm sure he would have made no dent in the deer population if he had run over Bambi. Plus, his car would not be as badly damaged if he had hit the deer properly.

For those that don't know, here is the proper way to hit a deer:
1. Turn your lights off so that it won't be blinded.
2. Honk your horn so that you may scare it off,
3. Speed up so that when you hit Rudolph, you send him flying. Otherwise, he'll roll up your hood, go through the windshield, and drive around giving you directions for the rest of the day.

So please, for the love of god and all that is good and pure, listen to this public service announcement: Just hit the damn animal. Unless it is your dog, or a small child in a Halloween costume, just hit it. You do a little damage to your car, and maybe piss off the dog owner, but you won't walk away with a collapsed lung and ruptured spleen like our friend.

Try this sometime for kicks: drinking Cherry Slurpees from 7-11 will always bring on a good trauma call.

Want to see an EMT blow his top? Wish him a quiet night.

Why are most of our patients healthier than we are?

Why do EDPs ask us if we think they are crazy? Is that an invitation to laugh in their face? Sometimes I feel like they are making some of this stuff up just to get a reaction out of us.

Did someone change the number on the side of my ambulance to 411? Why do people stop me in the middle of responding to a call, or on the scene, to ask for directions?

Here's a cure for this: give them wrong directions. Either give them the absolute longest way to get to where they're going, or just send them in the wrong direction. It may not stop people from asking for directions at the wrong time, but it sure will make you feel better.

Unless the patient is in a serious, life threatening emergency, the correct answer to the question "Will my insurance pay for this?" is NO. They will most likely sign a refusal after that.

Similarly, if, under the same circumstances, the question is "Will I be billed for this?" the answer is YES.

If your patient says that his or her ID is in the car and asks to go get it, let them. They will most likely drive off to avoid getting a bill. It's the old 'wallet in the car trick.'

When did rubbing alcohol become the miracle cure-all for Hispanic cultures?

The Great EMS Philosophical Debate: "If you hit a double-parked car while responding to a call and no one saw you, did you really hit it?"

There's one thing I don't understand (actually there are many things I don't understand but stay with me). Why does someone get hit by a car, or fall, or something along those lines, then walk up four flights of stairs, wait an hour to call, then expect me to carry them down? Why do they always have to make things harder than they need to be? Just leave them where they fall.

The lights on the top of your ambulance or fire truck have predictable effects on other drivers on the road. They will:
1. Suddenly become deaf and blind and not notice the big truck with all the flashing lights making all the noise,
2. Forget where they are, think they are a Nascar driver, and take off down the road.
3. Become so startled that they almost drive into the car in front of them or the concrete barrier next to them
4. Become so startled that they just stop right in front of you.
   But very few people pull to the right to get out of your way.

When responding to a call in heavy traffic, the sidewalk provides a much easier ride. More pedestrians to dodge, but hopefully less traffic.

From experience: When deciding to go the wrong way up a one way street, make sure it isn't a street that (A) your supervisor or chief of police lives on, or (B) is video taped by the local police.

The more serious the call you are going to, the less likely it will be that the other drivers on the road get out of your way.

The more BS the call, the more concerned the patient will be about how much time they have to spend in the ER.

Am I the only one who has had a patient take sleeping pills, then call an ambulance because they are feeling sleepy? I certainly hope not.

Heroin users crack me up. Why in God's name would you inject something into yourself that says right on the package things like DOA, Body Bag, or Fatal?

The scariest thing I ever heard was on the news. A child had just saved his father's life by doing CPR. He learned that from watching *Baywatch*. It kind of makes me worry about what else he picked up from the show. I wonder how long it will be before the kid is performing open-heart surgery with a ball point pen, defusing a bomb with a paper clip and a stick of gum, and making out with fake-breasted women all within the same hour.

I was reading a poster in an ER waiting room that listed some of the warning signs for teens at risk for suicide: irregular sleeping patterns, irregular appetite, feelings of being underappreciated, and hypersexuality. Strangely enough, that describes just about every EMT or Paramedic I have met.

Now that we have wonderful things like Enhanced 911 systems, radio identifiers, and global positioning for apparatus, can someone invent a BS detector for the 911 phone calls?

Better yet! Forget about AIDS or muscular dystrophy, can someone please come up with a cure for stupidity?

GREAT RADIO MOMENTS

It is impressed upon us that we are supposed to be professional at all times. Most importantly, we are supposed to be professional on the radio at all times because you never know who could be listening, including the FCC. But sometimes, situations present themselves and you just can't pass up the opportunity for a joke. Then there are the times when you just slip. These are some of the best things said over the radio.

"309 respond to Forest and Martin Luther King for . . . the man with absolutely nothing wrong with him. Says he wants to go to the hospital because he lives there."

"307 respond to the Engine 18 quarters. One of the firefighters there got some blood on him, and well . . . they want you to . . . actually I'm not sure what they want you to do. Just head over there."

"307 received and responding. Do you want me to stop at Walgreen's and pick up some soap?"

"304 respond to 921 Bergen Ave, on the outside, you can't miss it, car ran into a building."

"310, you're responding to 111 Leonard Street for the forty-six-year-old man who states that his skin is melting off because he hasn't had sex in several years."

"305 respond to 121 Delaware Ave, on the top floor, for an electrocution. Your cross street is Conduct Street, no pun intended."

"307 respond to 123 Congress Street for the baby that has been crying for the past two hours . . . your guess is as good as mine."

"311 respond to the corner of JFK Boulevard and Danforth for the man who done fell out."
"311 received. Ah, what did he fall out off?"
"He done fell out . . . the caller's words, not mine."

"310 to Dispatch. Can you call the police and have a radio car check on the EDP on the corner of Summit and Fairmount? He's brandishing a pretty big knife."
"310, we received. Can you give us a description of the person for the police?"
"A description? Sure look for the only guy standing in the middle of the street with a Crocodile Dundee knife in his hands."

"303 respond to the outside of 100 Westside Ave for the twenty-year-old female with pain in her rectum—I'll just leave it at that!"

"309 respond to 12 Carbon Street for the four-year-old with paper stuck in her nose. Yes, I said paper stuck in her nose."

"576 for the assignment. Respond to 2472 JFK Boulevard for the female who is coughing."

"Okay."

"576, from the caller, she states that it might—*might*—have something to do with the fact that her house is filling up with smoke."

"301 to Dispatch, did you receive my last transmission?"

"Ah, yeah . . . sorry. Someone must have given out the number for 911, and it's getting a little busy up here. Boy, if I find out who did that!"

"305 and 228, respond to 10 Exchange Place for the IP male on top of a limousine creating some type of disturbance."

"228, I'm in the area and there are a lot of limos here. Do you have anything further?"

"Sure, just look for the only drunk tap dancing on top of a limo."

"576, what's your location?"

"We're on the fourteenth floor of Progressive waiting for the elevator."

"Really, you're waiting for the elevator? Then how is it possible that the computer shows you are using your truck radio?"

"315 respond to 345 Corbin Street for the toothache. Let me know if you want the trauma team on standby."

"301 respond to 591 Montgomery for the seventy-four-year-old EDP."

"301 received. Should we wait for radio?"

"Well, she's seventy-four. I'm pretty sure you can take her if she gets violent."

"302 respond to 111 Storms Ave for the MVA [Motor

Vehicle Accident]. I'm assuming—and hoping—it's on the outside."

"305 respond to the rear of the Harborview Nursing Home. Someone tried to use the drive through window and found out there isn't one. Now his car is stuck in the side of the building."

"410, respond in North Bergen to the Palisades Nursing Home, room 315B for the confined cardiac arrest."
"410 to Dispatch, is that the nursing home that's attached to Palisades General Hospital?"
"That's affirmative."
"So let me get this straight. You're sending us to a hospital for a cardiac arrest? Sure, I can see that."

"311 to Dispatch, notify the ER we need the trauma team and are coming in with an unconscious stabbing patient. Patient was stabbed through the abdomen. Bleeding control measures initiated; patient on a long board and on high flow oxygen."
"311, we received. ER being notified. . . . The ER wants to know if the patient is having any trouble breathing."
"What? I don't know, he's unconscious, I asked him but he wouldn't answer me."

"Dispatch to 426, what's your status right now?"
"Single, no dependents."

"301, respond to the intersection of Pacific and Communipaw, at the payphone supposedly, for the . . . what? Is this a joke? Oh, you'll love this. Female with a condom stuck in her ear."

"305 to Dispatch, the E-squad wants to know how you

got this call before they force open the door to the person's house."

"Okay, 305, we got the call from Mobile Crisis who said that a deaf girl called them and said she was going to kill herself, which as I say sounds pretty weird because how would a deaf girl use the phone?"

"303, respond to 999 Rock Street for the animal bite."

"303 received. Is the animal under control?"

"The story is this: Jose called and said that Jose's dog bit Jose's kid and now Jose is going to blow the dog's head off. Police are getting reports of shots fired in the area, so you probably don't have to worry about Rover. Just use caution anyway."

A few minutes later . . .

"303, we're going to the hospital with one."

"305 to 303, how was the dog? . . . Well someone had to ask."

"302 to Dispatch, the patient was just sleeping. We woke him up and he walked away. We're back."

"Received, Rip Van Winkle is on his way."

"307, respond to Ocean and Bidwell, on the outside, for the man who states he is in cardiac arrest. I'm assuming your not gonna need paramedics, but keep me advised."

"305's arriving at the hospital, and put us out of service."

"What's the reason?"

"My patient says I have a little man hiding in my soap dispenser."

"309, you're responding for the IP male, laying on the sidewalk by Journal Square. The lady making the call says he looks like his face is melting off, so when you find out what that means, let me know."

"305, note the delay please. Instead of just buzzing us in like normal people would, the patient threw her keys at us. Now we have to figure out which one out of twenty is the right one."

"311, you'll be responding to 184 Cator Ave for the female with difficulty breathing. From the caller, and I don't know what to make of this, she's having trouble breathing because her mouth is twisted."

"416, what is your location?"
"My location? Well, that would be the exact spot I am in right now, but that's not important."
"Very funny, 416. I have a question for you."
"Sure, what's that?"
"A question? That's an interrogatory statement expressed for the purpose of gaining knowledge. But *that's* not important."

"305, respond to the Starlight Motel, room 35 for the female violent EDP."
"305 to Dispatch. I don't know what you've heard about me, but I don't frequent motels in this city. Can you give me an address?"

"307, respond to the intersection of Ravine and Palisades for the MVA."
"307 received. Can we get a cross street?"
"A what?"
"Can we get a cross street so we can find the call quicker?"
"Okay, rookie, let me walk you through this. The call location just so happens to be in an intersection. So, step one: take out your map. Step two: look up Palisades. Step three: run your finger up the page until you find Ravine. Step four:

drive to that location. There you will find an accident. If someone is hurt, then that is your call. That's simple enough, right?"

On the very next call:

"315, you'll be responding to the intersection of Summit and Sip for the MVA. Your cross streets will be Sip and Summit."

"576 to Dispatch. We've been in an accident, very minor, no injuries. Could you have the chief respond here?"

"Sure, what is your location?"

"We're at JFK and the Boulevard."

"Where are you?"

"JFK and the Boulevard."

"Where?"

(Very agitated) "JFK AND THE BOULEVARD!"

"Dispatch to 576, don't raise your voice, JFK *is* the Boulevard."

"310, respond to the outside of the bank on the corner of Bergen and JFK, for the man who says he is too drunk to walk."

"310 received. Ah, we're in the area and we don't see anything. Do you have a better location?"

"No, just look around. He said he was too drunk to walk, so I'm sure he couldn't have gotten far."

"305 to Dispatch. Be advised the first responders just informed us that the police said not to enter the scene until it is safe. So we'll be waiting outside."

"305, did they say why and are you in any danger?"

"No, they didn't say exactly why . . . only something about a domestic violence. I'm in no danger because I'm hiding in my truck down the street."

"Received. Duck and cover if you have to."

"225 for assignment. Chief, I need you to respond to Newkirk and Summit for the structure fire, with entrapment, with injuries, with jumpers, yadda, yadda, yadda, the whole nine yards."

"418, respond to 821 45th Street in North Bergen for the pronouncement. Actually, cancel that. We need you for a chest pain in Jersey City at 21 Rock Street.

"416, you'll respond for the pronouncement. 821 45th Street. On second thought, respond to the Wittpenn Bridge for the overturned vehicle.

"410, you'll respond, hopefully, for the pronouncement. You should know the address by now. 821 45th Street . . . Wait, no. Here we go again. You'll be responding to the asthma in Hoboken.

"224 to Dispatch. Will someone please handle that pronouncement sometime this summer before the body starts to decay!"

"428 to Dispatch, the bystanders are saying that this unconscious patient got up and was transported to the hospital by car. We'll be back."

"428, I need you to head to Ivy and Grand for another unconscious."

"Received." A few minutes later: "428, we'll be on scene. Patient is GOA as per the bystanders. Man, unconscious people sure get around in this city."

"304 to Dispatch, you can cancel the paramedics. This will be chest pains for the past two years."

"305 to Dispatch, notify FD that there is a dumpster fire on the corner of Kennedy and Broadman. We'll be standing by for them."

"305, why do you need to be there?"

"Because there's an idiot in flip-flops and shorts trying to stomp it out."

"Understood, sir."

"307, respond to the intersection of Summit and Magnolia for the man taking his clothes off, possibly waving at cars as he does so."

"414 to Dispatch, put this truck out of service. I think it's starting to overheat a little."

"The truck isn't on fire, is it, 414?"

"Ah, I can't really tell. There's too much smoke coming out of the hood. I'll try to make it back to the EMS garage."

"Received . . . No, wait! Get out of the truck now!"

"305 to Dispatch, give the ER a call and let them know we are coming in with a nineteen-year-old male, history of epilepsy, actively seizing."

"Do you have any vital signs?"

"No, I couldn't get one because he is still actively seizing."

"Oh, okay, I'm sure he'll stop eventually. One way or another."

"308 respond to 456 Duncan Ave for the pregnancy, female six years pregnant."

"Wait, did you say six years? Don't you mean six months?"

"No, she said six years. So either it's an EDP, or you better get there quick before she pops."

"315 to Dispatch. This truck is really starting to smoke now. We're gonna try to make to the hospital, then take us out of service."

"315, is that truck safe to drive?"

"Probably not."

"Well, okay, if you know what you are doing."

"I don't. Wish me luck."

"580 to Dispatch. Notify FD they have a working fire on the roof of the building in front of the [a city hospital]."

"580, we have to confirm that first."

"Confirm it? I know what fire looks like, and it's coming out of the roof of that building."

"311, respond to the K-Mart on Route 440. How tragic! A shoplifter was injured during his apprehension and he wants to go to the hospital. Huh, imagine that!"

"307 respond to 835 Bergen Ave for the . . . go over to Command for this one. [Command is a separate frequency so you don't tie up the primary channel. All the good information comes out on Command.] . . . You there? Okay, you're responding to the gentleman states he can't walk 'cause he has bugs on his feet."

"305, respond to the Dunkin Donuts on Summit Ave for the . . . well, you can go over to Command . . . You got the man who wants to go to the hospital because he needs a shower."

"A what?"

"Shower."

"As in a bath?"

"Yeah, now don't make me say it again."

"Okay, just ask the chief how we write this up because there's no check box on the report for cleanliness."

An hour later . . .

"305, I'm sorry for this. Respond to Beacon and Palisades, on the outside for the male, sick, unknown what his problem is. Actually, it's the same man you picked up from Dunkin Donuts, so I guess you do know what his problem is."

"309 to Dispatch, how did you get this EDP call?"

"The caller states that she thought she was being followed."

"Well, she said she was being followed because she WAS being followed."

I have a tendency to play music very loud while driving, and don't always turn the sound down when I use the radio. One day, I was listening to Isaac Hayes's "Theme from Shaft" a little too loud when I pulled up on scene.

"305's on scene."

"And we can dig it!"

On a radio report to the medical control doctor:

"428, we have a female patient, forty-nine years old, approximately 400 pounds. She's in cardiac arrest. We have an ETA to the hospital of about ten minutes once we get her out of her apartment."

"Repeat that weight for me please."

"Ah, 400 pounds . . . approximately."

"Would you like the forklift on standby?"

"Forklift? What is this, amateur comedy night?" [There actually is a forklift device in the ER that the paramedic didn't know about.]

"426 from Dispatch. The ER wants to know if that patient is stable."

"Uh, well, he's in cardiac arrest."

"Well, I guess you can't get more stabile than that."

"West 104, this will be a merchant-customer dispute. The john doesn't want to pay his hooker for services rendered. I can't believe she called us. We're taking them both in."—Jersey City Police Department

"Lawrence Control to Lawrence Ambulance, mutual aid to Lawrence Township . . ."

"Lawrence Control to Lawrence Ambulance, respond to the Quakerbridge Mall for the possible broken hand."
"Ambulance received and responding for the hand job . . . err, sorry."

After discovering that their pedestrian struck was actually a deer hit by a car:
"Lawrence Ambulance to Lawrence Control, Bambi signed the refusal. We'll be back in service."

"Eagles' Chase Command from Central. The caller states that her carbon monoxide detector is going off. She said she started her car and left the garage door closed. Went into the house and did some laundry while the car warmed up. Then the alarm started going off."
"And she's now wondering why her alarm is going off? Tell her to open the door."

"Ewing ambulance to Central, we're receiving gunfire on the corner of Calhoun and Martin Luther King."
"If you are in danger, leave the area."
"Are you kidding? My momma didn't raise no dummy, I'm heading home!"

"Engine 1, Ladder 1, Rescue 1, North Battalion [Trenton FD], respond to 12 Calhoun Street for either a suicidal jumper or a psychiatric emergency."
"North Battalion received. Do you have description on the party?"
"Yes. He's the person climbing around on the outside of the building dressed as Superman."

(On a paramedic report to a doctor) "12 X-Ray, doc, listen up and listen good, 'cause I'm only gonna say this once! We're coming in with a thirty-four-year-old male, hypotension secondary to an eggplant being lodged in his rectum."

"11 Z, note to hospital 20. Five minutes out, asthmatic male, BP of 120/80, 84 pulse, 18 respirations. ALS on board."
(From Dispatcher) "Hospital notified, five minutes out, with a perfectly healthy male, they're waiting. Stop wasting my time."

"Attention all units, a signal 10-75 [working fire] has been announced in the Borough of Queens, address is 31–38 78th Street"
(A frantic voice on the radio from an unknown unit) "Jesus Christ, that's my house."
"Really?"
"No, not really."

"11 Z to Central, I think I know where we are going. Up Lenox Ave, make a left at 16 V's ambulance on the corner doing nothing, and the call should be five blocks up on the right."
"Okay, in that case, Central to 16 V for the assignment . . ."

"Central to 11 Patrol. Can I get an update on the fire?"
"11 Patrol with an update: Three story warehouse, lots of smoke, lots of fire, lots of people running in and out with hoses."

"Central to 12 V, can I get an update on your status? You've been 40 minutes in the ER?"
"Okay, 12 V to Central, now it's 41 minutes in the ER."

"16 D to Central, put a rush on PD, I'm in no danger, but I really need the handcuffs to get this EDP to the hospital."

"Central to 16 D, what's the problem, then?"

"Well . . ."

(In the background from the patient) "JESUS LOVES YOU, BUT I'M GONNA KICK YOUR CRACKER ASS!"

"Central to 16 D, we received that directly."

After several alert tones:

"16 D, you have an assignment, please acknowledge."

"16 D to Central, send it again there's nothing on my MDT."

"Central to 16 D, I didn't send it yet, I figured I would wake you up first."

"12V from Central. We have further information on your asthma patient. She is actually a violent EDP. Use caution."

"Well, thank you, but I became painfully aware of that when she came charging down the hall trying to kill me!"

(New York Police Department Dispatcher) "Three males with weapons on the corner of Lenox and 125th. Perpetrators are two white males, blue jeans, Rangers jerseys. One black male, Yankee jersey, and baseball cap. All armed with pistols."

"Sector David, Central, you just described our undercover unit."

"Oh, you're right, sorry. Disregard that then."

WORKING CODE

The lobby of the nursing home is deserted. There is not even a receptionist to greet us as we come through the door. *Of course there isn't; there's never one when you need her.* I call the dispatcher and double check the floor. My dispatcher tells me he thinks it's the fourth floor. *Great! He thinks?* After my extremely rocky start, the day has started to shape up. Sure, we were busy, but nothing major has happened in the last three hours. That's a good sign, *I hope.*

We squeeze into the elevator and head for the fourth floor. As we step off the elevator, my partner comments to me that everyone on the floor seems too calm to have someone in cardiac arrest. "There should be at least one nurse running around like a chicken with her head cut off," he says. *Very good point.*

I ask the nurse at the nurses' station if someone is in cardiac arrest. She says, "No, try the third floor."

Grumbling and cursing, we head back for the elevator. We get off on the third floor and we get the same feeling that these people are just too quiet. I ask the nurse at the nurses' station if they have someone in cardiac arrest. She tells me no. Luckily, as we head for the elevator, the stereotypical frantic nurse comes running out of the room yelling to the head nurse for some equipment. This was the right floor. *How can the lady at the front desk* not *know someone is in cardiac arrest on her floor?* There's no time to find out the answer for that.

Inside the room, the nurses still have the patient on the bed, doing CPR on him. They are doing compressions but I can see from across the room that they are ineffective. Every time they push on his chest, the patient bounces up and down on the bed. As I get closer, I see that, instead of doing ventilations with a bag valve mask (with which you force air into the lungs) they have a regular oxygen mask on the patient. I guess they are hoping that oxygen trickles down the man's throat.

The first thing I do is to move the patient onto the floor. I check for a pulse and don't find one. I resume CPR while my partner attaches the defibrillator to the patient. I stop what I am doing and back away when I hear the automated voice from the machine say loudly, "Stand clear! Stand clear!" My partner yells for everyone to clear. Not that it was necessary for him to do so since most of the nurses have left us alone with the patient. As the machine is analyzing the patient's heart rhythm, the paramedics arrive. The machine says once more, "Stand clear! Stand clear!" This time it is followed by a high-pitched wail from the defibrillator as it charges up to deliver a shock.

"Everyone clear?" My partner calls out as he looks around the patient to double check. Everyone backs up a step.

The voice from the machine calls out, "Press to shock! Press to shock!" My partner does one more check to make sure everyone is clear. Then he presses the button to deliver the shock.

There is a *fwump* sound. The patient's chest jumps off

the ground in a convulsive fit. In the fit, his arm swings out and hits my partner in the leg, transferring some of the electricity into him. My partner doesn't go down, merely jumps back and stands up.

We begin to work on the patient. A few minutes later, as we are getting ready to leave for the hospital, my partner finally asks, "Should I be having chest pains?"

Absolutely terrific! My partner just defribrillated himself! Why me?

FUN WITH DOAs AND ODs

As insensitive as it sounds, it is all right to laugh a little when dealing with death. One of the best ways to cope with the stresses of the job, I've found, is to find something funny at the scene and laugh about it later. It's never good to laugh at the person, or even to laugh while on scene, but sometimes, things will happen that you will just find funny.

I was dispatched for an unconscious female. When we arrived on scene, a group of young children—the oldest was about twelve—came running out of the house towards us. All four of them were crying or screaming. When I asked what happened, they told me their grandmother wouldn't wake up. I asked them to show me the way and they took off upstairs.

Upstairs, a twelve year old girl was on the phone, crying hysterically, with her grandmother lying face down on the bed. I had a strong feeling that the grandmother was already dead. My feeling was confirmed when my partner and I rolled her onto the floor and her body maintained the same position, rigid with rigor mortis.

My heart immediately went out to the children. The look in their eyes told me all I needed to know: their grandmother was someone they loved deeply. I would imagine that she was the only mother figure these children had.

I feel no shame in admitting that my eyes were welling up with tears. Thankfully, though, as I was fighting back that feeling, the girl said a lady on the phone wanted to talk to me. Thinking it was a family member, I nervously took the phone. Dealing with family members of the deceased is never an enviable job. "Hello?" I asked.

"Hello," a voice called back. "911, what is your emergency?"

"What?" I was stunned for a moment. "Oh, no emergency, this is the ambulance."

"What?" the voice crowed back. "You need an ambulance?"

"No, this is the EMS."

"What? You want to talk to the EMS?"

My god, woman! Clean out your ears! Your job is to listen, and you're not listening to me! I get a little laugh out of that every time I think about that day. It sucked to have to look at the kids and not be able to do anything to help. But, thankfully, I have that oh-so-efficient dispatcher to laugh at.

Another time I can remember being upset by my job happened when some sanitation workers made a gruesome discovery. While doing the rounds very early in the morning, some workers discovered a baby laying on one of the conveyer belts in the sewer treatment plant.

We were dispatched to check on the baby because the workers had not yet gotten to it to see if it was still alive. When we arrived, we realized right away from the bloatedness and discoloration that the baby was dead. Sad as that seems, it got worse.

Our first reaction was that the baby may have fallen into the sewer somehow and accidentally drowned. *I wish that were what happened.* As we got closer to the body, we saw that the umbilical cord was still attached. Some monster gave birth to the child and dumped her into the sewer. I know it's harsh to call the person a monster because I don't know her situation. However, if you had seen this gruesome site, you would understand why I can't think of any other way to describe the mother.

This might have driven me completely crazy, had it not been for the circumstances that preceded the discovery. My partner and I were right around the corner from the treatment plant relaxing. It was very early in the morning, I believe it was around 3 AM, and we were tired, so we were taking turns napping. My partner was asleep and I was reading a book when nature decided to call. *And when nature calls, I pick up the phone.*

We were in the middle of nowhere, so I figured it would be alright to step out and do my business in the bushes. As I was standing there, a sanitation truck drove down the street towards the treatment plant. It made me jump a little, but I didn't think anything of it until it paused in front of the ambulance for a moment. The driver made some sort of gesture, which I later found out was him trying to get me to follow him. I thought he was getting mad at me for urinated in the bushes. He drove off, then I went back to the truck.

As I climbed back in, I heard on the radio that the dispatcher was sending the chief to the sewer treatment plant around the corner from where I was because the workers "found something" and they needed to talk to him about it. I nearly wet myself, thinking they had called to report me for urinating in the bushes and my partner for sleeping. I woke him up, and we both sat in the truck panicking. We were so scared that we would lose our jobs. Just before we burst into tears, however, the dispatcher called for a paramedic unit and an ambulance to respond to the scene.

It was that moment when I thought my job was on the line because I got in touch with nature that always brings the right amount of levity to the situation when I think about it.

I was sitting around the first aid squad one Sunday morning watching the twenty-four-hour marathon of Scooby Doo cartoons. *What can I say? I'm easily amused.* I had the fire/police scanner on and I was listening to what was going on in the county. One of the township's fire companies was dispatched to a supermarket for a tractor-trailer on fire. I heard the captain call frantically on the radio. "Captain 21 to Central. We need an ambulance out here now! There's someone entrapped in a car under the truck!"

I was in the ambulance with the engine running before the dispatcher called us. When we arrived on scene, we found that a car had driven lengthwise under a parked trailer. The car looked like it had driven between the upright stands of the trailer and was now lying completely under the trailer. I could see a body slumped over the wheel, not moving.

No one had check for a pulse yet, and somehow that became my job. I crawled under the tractor-trailer, the whole time thinking, *This doesn't seem too safe!* I found that the patient had a very faint pulse.

"All right, it's not safe under there. Now get out of there before the trailer collapses on you." *Gees, thanks for telling me now! I would have liked to have been told that little tidbit BEFORE I crawled under there.*

It took some time before we could stabilize the trailer, but when we did, guess who had to go back in and hold stabilization on the head. First I needed to find a way to get into the vehicle. The firefighters were saying that they had to pry open the doors because they couldn't open any of them, but something made me want to look for myself.

I walked around to the passenger side door. I could reach the door without placing myself in any danger, and I tried the door. It wouldn't open, just like they said. But something made me look again. The window was broken and I could see the door was still locked. I unlocked the door, and let myself in.

"How did you do that?" the astonished captain asked.

"I guess I just have the hands of life."

I slipped into the vehicle and checked for a pulse again. There was no pulse now. Seeing that it might be awhile before they extricated the patient, I shifted myself to get comfortable. "Scott!" I called to partner, almost crying.

"Devin, what's up?"

"Doing me a favor," with a quiver in my voice. "Count how many fingers he has."

"Okay, um there's ten. Why?"

"See if maybe he's missing a piece of his ear or something."

"No he's not. Look, what is going on?"

"Scott. What the hell did I just sit on?" Jumping out of the car and looking down, I saw that I was sitting on a chunk of his brains. Sometimes, when he needs a good laugh, Scott will turn to me and say, "What the hell did I just sit in?"

One night, the first aid squad was dispatched for an MVA with entrapment. I hopped in the car and responded from home. The accident was on the road that I take to get to squad, and since I wouldn't be able to get around it, I went to the scene.

A car had been traveling down Route 206, probably at a high rate of speed. As it came upon a curve, the driver must have wiped out due to the snow that was falling. His car jumped up onto the grass, flipped on its side, and continued to travel about 25 feet and wrap itself around a utility pole.

There was one patient in the car, and he had a slight

pulse. Unfortunately, there was no easy way to get the patient out of the car. We would have to winch the car away from the pole, then cut the roof off, and finally remove the patient. The operation lasted around a half an hour, during which the patient went into cardiac arrest.

We managed to remove the patient and saw that there was nothing we could have done to save him. His ribs were broken in several places, his legs were both broken at the tibia and fibula, kneecaps were shattered, and back was broken in several places. He had hit the steering wheel so hard that his face had left an impression in the center of the wheel. The paramedic assessing him was pointing out all of his injuries like a child. "Hey guys look at this! Wow, his back isn't supposed to bend like that. This is cool!"

The patient was turned over to the ME, and we finished cleaning up. I walked back to my car in the rapidly increasing snow. There was about an inch of powder on the ground. I learned a very important lesson then: *No one carries jumper cables.*

I forgot to unplug my blue light and it drained my car battery. The ambulance didn't have cables, neither did the fire truck, the police, not even the tow truck! I had to sit in the freezing car and radio for our Captain to go back to his house to pick up some cables. Finally, two VERY cold hours later, my car was driveable again. People still remind me when I show up at a scene to make sure my blue light is off.

I was dispatched to assist another crew with CPR in Jersey City one night. As I was walking up the stairs, one broke and I almost fell through. That is never a good sign. When we got upstairs, I saw the other crew doing CPR on a very large man. I could see that they were tired already, so I took over compressions.

The man just went into cardiac arrest on them, so they hadn't had the chance to put the defibrillator on him yet. I stopped compressions while they put on the pads and I set up the Reeves. I said over my shoulder, "Pedro, he's got a really hairy chest, you'll need to shave him." Now, when you shave someone for defib, you just have to take a razor and shave off patches. Doesn't have to be neat, and you can just dry shave because he's not going feel anything anyway.

I didn't pay much attention when I heard the soft 'pop' followed by a swirling sound. I turned my attention back to doing CPR and saw Pedro shaving the patient, but with a mound of shaving cream on his chest. "What are you doing?" the paramedic yelled. "That cream is alcohol based; it'll catch fire when you shock him!" We frantically rubbed off the cream, put the pads on, and defibrillated him a few times with no fire.

We loaded him onto the Reeves, just barely able to strap him in, and attempted a six-man carrying down the stairs. (*Not my idea. I was the FNG and no one would listen to me when I voiced my reservations.*) As we carried him down the stairs, the steps broke on me again, and this time I got my foot stuck. We managed to get him to the hospital without injuring ourselves any further.

Afterwards, we were all talking outside of the ER, and Pedro walked out to join us. We all stopped talking, and the paramedic turned to him and said, "I have one VERY important question for you: where'd ya get the shaving cream?"

The Fire Department of Jersey City was dispatched as the first responders for a person with difficulty breathing. When they arrived on scene, the family informed the firefighters that the patient just had the flu. However, when they looked at her, they found the patient was stiff as a board and showing signs of obvious death.

The captain ordered the firefighters to begin CPR just for the sake of the family. As they were doing CPR, one of the firefighters noticed that the family members were leaning over, almost trying to look around him. He didn't think anything of it, and continued compressions. He looked up again a few minutes later, and they were still looking at him funny, like they were trying to look behind him.

Finally, he looked up a third time and noticed them doing this. He turned around to see what they were looking at. The TV was on behind him, and the family was trying to watch it while they were doing CPR.

On another occasion, FDJC was dispatched as the first responders for an unconscious/unresponsive patient lying in the street. When they arrived, there was a man sitting on the side of the street. Some of his friends were jumping up and down waving for the fire truck. The patient was dazed, and his pants were soaked.

One of his friends informed the firefighters that the young man had probably overdosed on heroin. So, in their infinite wisdom, they thought it would be beneficial to open the man's pants and dump snow down them to try to wake him up. That didn't work quite like they had in mind, so they called 911.

When the ambulance and paramedics arrived, they began to give the man Narcan and an IV. During the process of giving the man the IV, he bled a little more than they expected. Not thinking anything of it, the crew wiped up the blood with guaze pads and set them down on the man's stomach. They intended to throw them away when they were done.

When the Narcan was administered, the patient woke up. He saw the bloody gauze pads on his stomach. "What's that?" he asked pointing at the mess.

Not missing a beat, the sympathetic paramedic said, "Oh yeah, that. Well, when we found you, there was some big brother sodomizing you. That's the packing we plugged your bleeding asshole with."

"No! You're not serious, are you?" The man was in tears.
"You don't believe me? Are your balls wet?"
"Yu-yes."
"Then why don't you believe me?"

I hope that was enough to get the man into rehab, but probably not.

I thought it was pretty funny the first time I heard that people stuff ice down the pants of a heroin OD. Yet, to my surprise, it seems to be a pretty common practice, or maybe just for FDJC.

An engine company was returning from a fire alarm one evening when they were flagged down by a frantic female. She was saying that her boyfriend had overdosed on heroin and he wasn't waking up.

The captain radioed for an ambulance and they went in to investigate. The man was waking up by the time they made it upstairs. He was sitting up in the bed and seemed more concerned about why his pants were undone than why the firefighters were in his house.

The front of his pants were wet, and he reached in to feel around. He pulled out an uncooked chicken leg. He studied it for a moment, then put it on the table. He reached in, then pulled out another chicken leg, then another, and finally one more.

All proud of herself, the wife said, "I couldn't find any ice, so I just threw some frozen chicken down his pants." She looked away from the stunned firefighters toward her husband. "Hey, honey, now that them legs are defrosted, you wanna have chicken for dinner?"

"Yeah," he said, "chicken legs sound good!"

An ambulance was dispatched to a construction site in Jersey City for an unconscious patient. The patient was on the seventh floor of a building under construction, and only one small freight elevator was operating. The patient was a big man. 'Big' as in a strong man. He must have had one massive heart attack, because from all accounts he went right out.

The crew started CPR and asked what his name was. The foreman told him it was Rocky. So one of the EMTs began to talk to the patient, like many of us do. It's sort of a subconscious thing, like maybe if we talk to him, he'll come back. So he's bent over the patient, doing compressions, saying softly, "Ah, come on, Rocky."

Everyone else at the site must have picked up on it, because they began to start yelling, "Come on, Rocky! Come on, Rocky!" like he was fighting Apollo Creed. All of the workers had stopped working and were now hanging on the rafters like the fight scene in *Mad Max Beyond Thunderdome*.

The paramedics showed up and made the determination that they would have to lower him in a basket from the seventh floor. They called in the fire department and began work on starting IVs and intubating the patient. The medic was having a hard time putting the tube in and yelled to his partner, "Gene, you'll have to do this, he's not taking the tube."

Suddenly, there was hush over the crowd. The foreman got down on one knee, shook his fist in the air at the patient and cheered him on: "Take the tube, Rock, take the tube." Then everyone else joined in. "Take the tube, Rock, Take the tube."

By this time, one of the EMTs had begun to whistle "Eye of the Tiger" loud enough for his partner and the medic to hear. Fighting back laughter, they went about defibrillating the patient. After twenty (yes, *twenty*) shocks and a pharmacy's worth of medications, they got a pulse back. There was a loud cheer and applause from the workers. The EMT whistling turned to the medics and began saying, "Adrian, Adrian, I did it!"

★ ★ ★

A crew in Jersey City was dispatched for an unconscious, possibly not breathing. When they arrived, they found the patient was breathing but had a faint pulse. He had pinpoint pupils, fresh needle tracks on his arm, and heroin works sitting on the counter. The paramedics arrived and began to treat the patient.

The patient's friends didn't speak much English and were starting to get in the way, so one of the paramedics had them hold hands and sing 'Amazing Grace.' As they sang, his partner gave the patient Narcan, which counters the heroin. The first dose didn't work, so he told the friends to sing harder as they gave him more Narcan. When the patient sprung to life, kicking and swinging, they all began to rejoice and sang louder.

I arrived on scene for a heroin overdose to find a man was performing mouth-to-mouth on the patient. This would have been a good thing, if the patient wasn't already breathing on his own. "I did mouth to mouth!" the proud man said.

"You did? Oh no . . ." I was about to say that wasn't really necessary because the patient was already breathing, but one of the paramedic's cut me off.

"Dude, you gave him mouth-to-mouth? Well, he's breathing—that means you're gay." He said that with such a serious look on his face that the man believed him.

"Oh no, I ain't gay!" He was almost in tears trying to deny it.

After giving the patient some Narcan, he woke up. While he was still coming to, his wife walked down the hallway. "Is this your husband, ma'am?" I asked her. She answered me, but it was an unintelligible mumble. She looked like she had been spiking up with her husband. Still being serious, I asked her what her husband's name was. She mumbled again.

"Now we're getting somewhere!" the chief yelled to me with a smile from across the room.

"So ma'am," I asked her straight faced and loud enough so that the paramedics could hear me. "Does your husband do heroin?" The paramedics, who were trying hard to start an IV, burst into laughter.

"No, no. Devin, you got the wrong guy," they yelled to me. "The needle tracks, pin point pupils, the response to Narcan; no, he don't do heroin!"

We were having way too much fun. We loaded the patient in the ambulance and took him to the hospital. While en route, the man's mumbling wife sat up front with me. I pulled into the parking lot of the hospital, less than a half a mile from the man's house, and told her we were here. I got out without looking at her. When I walked around to the back of the truck, I noticed she was still in the front seat.

"Can you see if she's okay?" I asked the chief. "Maybe she needs some Narcan too."

"My wife doesn't do drugs!" the man yelled to us as we pulled him out.

She doesn't do drugs, eh? She was passed out in the front seat of the ambulance, probably from the same heroin he was doing.

An ambulance in Ewing, New Jersey, was dispatched one evening for an unknown emergency. A police car had spotted a man laying on the side of the road and asked for an ambulance without checking it.

No sooner did the ambulance sign on the air that they were responding than the police unit came over the radio screaming for a rush and that the patient didn't have a pulse. The ambulance responded to that by screaming on the EMS channel to the dispatcher for a paramedic unit.

So now everyone started going crazy, yelling, "I'm closer to that"—"No, I'm closer!" I can only imagine the dispatcher's head spinning trying to keep up with all the units speaking on the radio.

The ambulance arrived on the scene, announcing themselves by screaming into the radio. The dispatcher told them to get an update as soon as they can. They came back yelling for the paramedics to come down such-and-such a street. Then, after a long, drawn out pause, the ambulance comes back on the radio and tells the dispatcher to cancel everyone. Not stopping there, I guess wanting to embarrass themselves further, the crew admits on the radio that this was just a mannequin that someone threw away.

I was called to a nursing home in Jersey City for a cardiac arrest. The patient had been in cardiac arrest for a few minutes before we got there, and the staff had begun CPR. We took over, began defibrillation, and packaged her to go to the hospital. The paramedics showed up, started IVs, and worked their magic, but she was still in cardiac arrest when we loaded her into the ambulance.

The nursing home was right around the corner from the hospital so we were there in a minute. She was still in cardiac arrest when we started to wheel the stretcher out of the truck. For some unknown reason, the stretcher's wheels did not catch, and we dropped the stretcher. It bounced off the floor of the ambulance, then bounced off the back step, then bounced once when it hit the ground. Miraculously, we looked at the monitor and she had regained a rhythm and a pulse. Luckily, no one saw us drop her. *Yeah we brought her back, but that's not a move I think the American Heart Association would endorse.*

I was on a call with my brother Sean in Lawrenceville for a pedestrian struck. It was in the middle of US Route 1 in front of a busy diner and a welfare motel. The commotion of the police cars and ambulance had attracted the attention of the people inside both places. Inside the motel they were knocking on each other's doors, getting everyone out to take a look at what was going on.

The patient was bleeding badly from somewhere, but we couldn't see the injury. The medics told Sean to cut the man's shirt off and see if he was bleeding from somewhere on his chest.

Sean cut the shirt off, and was instantly made aware of the man's punctured carotid artery when the blood shot out of his neck and all over Sean's shirt. Suddenly there was a horrified scream: "He just slit that man's throat. Oh my God!" Then everyone began screaming and passing out.

An ambulance was dispatched to a senior citizen's center for a possible cardiac arrest. When they arrived, the crew found that the gentleman was several days past his expiration. They notified the dispatcher, who then reassigned the paramedics for another call. The tour chief decided she would respond over to the senior center to relieve the crew until the paramedics could come back and make the pronouncement.

The crew thought they would have a little fun with the chief. When she walked in the room, the crew was saying, "Okay, sir, just sign here. If you have anymore problems, just call again." And to accent it, they picked up the man's arm and dropped it on the refusal sheet, making a scribble mark where he should sign his name.

Dumbfounded, the chief just looked at them and said, "You guys ain't right."

NURSING HOME NIGHTMARES

"Good afternoon, ma'am. How are you today?" I asked with a smile as I walked into her room.

"I'm fine. Who are you?"

"My name is Devin; I'm with the transportation service. We're here to take you to [a nursing facility in Jersey City]. You'll like it there; the people are very friendly."

"That sounds very nice . . . what is this place? Is it another hospital?"

"No, ma'am, it's a nursing home."

"It's a WHAT? WHO TOLD YOU TO BRING ME THERE?"

"Umm, I believe it was your son?"

"That bastard, where is he? I'm gonna kill him!"

There was a time when I feared dying, when I wanted so badly to grow old and gray. Those days are long since gone for me because I have seen what lies ahead for me, and it ain't pretty. I'm not sure if karma exists, but I have a funny feeling that the things I do today will catch up to me later. I know that, because I tell these stories, I am going to wind up living out my Golden Years in one of these nursing homes.

When people think of a nursing home, they usually think of a quiet place where someone can get quality care. But, like UFOs, I have heard these types of places exist but I've never seen them.

A great thing about nursing calls is that you never know what sort of people you will encounter when you go there. There's a lady in a nursing home in Jersey City who walks around to all of the visitors, licking her gums and drooling at the mouth and asking, "You wanna get lucky? You wanna get some?"

There was a gentleman in a nursing home in Lawrenceville who would constantly masturbate. I mean he would continuously fondle himself all day long—never finish, just play with himself. And the great part was that the geniuses at the nursing home gave him the room that faced the visitors' elevator. So everyone who came to visit was treated to the sight of this man in all his glory.

If I don't manage to grow old gracefully and need to be placed in a nursing home, I want someone to just give enough food to last a few days, and then dump me in the middle of nowhere. Hell, it worked for nomadic tribesmen; why not me?

In Lawrenceville, we have a very prominent rehabilitation center/nursing home. Hospitals from all over New Jersey send their patients there be rehabilitated after an accident or debilitating illness. The rehabilitation center impresses me. If I ever get hurt, I'd like to go there. The nursing care facility scares the living crap out of me.

Part of the reason is that, from an EMS responder's point of view, I have noticed that the nature of the dispatch rarely matches up with the real call. Case in point:

We were dispatched there one morning for a "Cardiac

Arrest, CPR in progress." So we respond over there, placing the other motorists and ourselves on the road in danger. We grab all the equipment off the truck, race upstairs, run into the room, get ready for business, and what do we find?

"Nice of you guys to show up. I'm an hour late for my appointment." There he was, sitting in a chair watching Sunday morning church services on the TV, and as alive as you or me.

"They do nice work here," I said, "sort of like on *Baywatch* but without the hot women."

We double-checked the room number, then walked down the hall to see if anyone was dead (since no one spoke up, I guessed they were okay). "Can I help you?" the nurse at the nursing station asked.

"Of course you can. Who's in cardiac arrest?" my brother Sean asked.

"No one that I know of. Who called?"

"Obviously someone on this floor. We don't come here for our health."

"I called, but I didn't say anything about CPR. I just wanted to see if you could transport him."

"Well someone did. I know some of our dispatchers are idiots, but even they can't screw this up."

So we had the dispatcher pull the 911 tape, and sure enough, the caller was screaming into the phone that the patient was in cardiac arrest.

Don't be fooled into thinking that only happens at one facility. An ambulance was dispatched to another nursing home for "CPR in Progress." When the crew arrived on scene, they were greeted at the elevator by an orderly. He was sporting an ear to ear grin. "He was in cardiac arrest. I did CPR and I brought him back." He was so proud of himself.

"That's wonderful, sir," the driver said. "Where is the patient?"

They were directed to the patient's room; where much to their surprise, the patient was up and walking around. They were taken aback for a moment because, unless you are on *Baywatch*, people do not get up and walk around after CPR.

They decided they better talk to the head nurse. Not surprisingly, after what they saw in the room, the nurse had no idea why they were even there. And even less surprising, they couldn't find the orderly anywhere.

The disturbing thing about this is not that he could have lied about the patient being in cardiac arrest, but that he may have actually been doing compressions on a live patient. I wouldn't put it past him.

I used to do inter-facility transports in Jersey City. We would take people from a hospital to nursing homes or other hospitals. My partner at the time had some stories ...

One day he was taking a patient to a nursing home in the Newark, New Jersey, area. While he was waiting for the staff to register the patient, another patient approached him. She was rubbing herself all over, and saying, "Gimme the cheese, baby, gimme the cheese!"

"Sorry, ma'am, I don't have any cheese." And he turned to his partner. "What the heck is she talking about?"

Thinking nothing of it, they went about their business. They moved their patient into her room, and the lady from before approached them again. "Gimme the cheese, baby, you gotta gimme the cheese."

"Okay, maybe I'll give you the cheese later," he said.

They moved the patient over, handed in the paperwork, and got ready to leave. "Gimme the cheese, baby, you gotta give me the cheese." This time, she was rubbing herself and wiggling her hips.

"What the hell are you talking about?"

"Gimme the cheese, baby, I wanna see you cum!"
AAAAAAHHHHHH!!!! I feel violated writing about it.

The one thing I always get a kick out of is how feisty many older women are. I've had more propositions from old women than I have from women my own age. I had a patient that I took to dialysis on a regular basis. She looks like a black Yoda. She's about three feet tall and balding, with patches of gray hairs sprouting from her chin. She has round, lizard-like eyes (*no pun intended*) that never open more than a slit, and her bottom lip is always pouting like she is about to say something. Her voice is so shrill, like nails grating against the chalkboard. And she never speaks, only yells.

Her problem is that she has lost her mind. She thinks my name is Tito. There is no way I look anything like a Tito. I was Tito, and my partner James was Virginia. I guess Virginia and Tito were the last people to take her to dialysis before she lost her mind.

I hear that voice in my sleep at night: "TITO, gimme my tissues! TITO, drive slow or I'm gonna throw up! If you don't pull my leg down, I'm gonna start biting!"

One day, we were waiting for the elevator in a crowded lobby. She mumbled something to me, but because of the noise in the lobby, I couldn't hear her. "What's that?" So she mumbled it again. The noise seemed to increase this time when I asked. Maybe that was the signal to stop asking, but of course I didn't listen. "What?"

Of course, all the noise stops as soon as she yells out her answer. "TITO, I'm horny, get in the bed. Come on Tito, get in the bed." *WOW, what a smoothie she is. Clear the way, momma, I'm coming in.*

"Fanny, you know you shouldn't say things like that."

"COME ON, TITO, I love ya, just a little kiss. I love ya, Tito!"

There's really no cool way to cover it up when a sixty-seven-year-old is demanding sex from you in front of a crowd of people waiting for an elevator.

I was called to a nursing facility in Lawrenceville one night for a cardiac arrest. The staff had rolled the patient into the corner of the room, and there were about three really small nurses trying to work on this really big man. "All right, guys, back up, let us through." My partner said. We got in there and began CPR after assessing that he really was in cardiac arrest.

"Let's pull him out into the middle of the room so we have more room to work. Devin, grab his feet." I grabbed ahold of his enormous legs, not noticing that one was slightly different than the other, and I yanked. *Cccrrack!*

"Holy shit!" I screamed, almost in tears, as I held one lose limb in my hands. "I think I broke his leg."

Everyone got a good laugh out of my anguish before they told me I ripped of his wooden leg. Here I am thinking I yanked the guy's leg out of its socket. I'm just glad that everyone gets such amusement from my pain.

CPR calls in a nursing home are always fun because, like an EDP, you never know what you're going to find. I responded to one at the same nursing home and found the staff doing compressions, but no ventilations. I'm sorry, let me correct that: they had the patient on 2 liters of oxygen through a nasal cannula. So the patient would be getting oxygenated air IF the patient could breathe. And the kicker was that they were proud that they thought to put the patient on oxygen. Well, they get a gold star in my book, I guess.

On another occasion, I was driving home from the store when I heard over my volunteer pager that there was a cardiac arrest at the nursing home. A wave of civic duty rushed over me—I decided to lend a hand. I was right at the intersection in front of the nursing home, so I went there. I found a phone, called the first aid squad, and told them to meet me at the scene. I decided that I would head upstairs and make sure that this was, in fact, a cardiac arrest and not someone late for their proctologist's appointment.

I walked into the room, wearing a first aid squad jacket that clearly identified me as a member of the township's first aid squad and told them who I was. And the nurse still asked me, "Are you family?"

"No, I'm not family. Didn't you listen to anything I just said?"

"Oh, you're from the squad. Well, we have everything under control. You can step back for now." I looked in and saw what they called under control: the defibrillator cart was in the hallway, there were six nurses around him and no one touching him, the bag-valve-mask (or AmbuBag for those who watch ER) was laying beside his head, the nursing supervisor was pulling the EKG leads off of his clothes (for those who don't know, the E.G. leads don't go on the clothes, they're supposed to go on the skin), one nurse was pulling the sheet over the patient's head, and another nurse was saying, "Do you want me to call Doctor So-and-So to get the pronouncement?"

So, for those playing along at home, what can we logically infer from this scene? Most people would assume that the nursing staff has called it and the patient is dead.

That's what I thought at least. So I asked the nursing supervisor, "Does this mean what I think it means?"

"We have everything under control."

"Yes, but does this mean you are calling it."

"We have everything under control." *What the hell, am I talking to a parrot? Do you know any words other than that?*

I walked out of the room and canceled the paramedics, and told the ambulance to slow down their response but to keep coming to get the patient information.

A few minutes later, the ambulance arrived, and the nursing supervisor came out of the room and asked, "Are the paramedics still coming?"

"No, I canceled them."

"You did WHAT?!" And she proceeded to yell at me in the hallway, in front of staff and patients.

"Listen, if you have a problem with what I did, let's discuss this in private and not in front of everyone." So we went into her office and she continued to berate me.

"What gives you the right? How dare you? Who says you can cancel the paramedics?"

Feeling cocky, I looked at the EMT patch on the jacket, then at her, then back at the patch, and said, "State of New Jersey." That seemed to infuriate her even more and she kept on yelling.

"I am the nursing supervisor, and I am the higher medical authority in this facility, so you listen to me."

"Well, I asked you several times if you were calling it, and you said you had everything under control. Since you said that, and no one was doing anything, I assumed that you had called the patient."

"Don't you tell me we weren't doing CPR."

"You guys weren't doing anything for the patient. I've been an EMT for four years. I know that when you are not touching the patient, the defib is in the hall, and you are pulling a sheet over the patient's head, you ain't doing anything."

"That's not true. I have been a nursing supervisor for the last ten years and—"

"I guess what you are saying is that you found a new way to do CPR?"

It took her a few seconds to register that, but then she started yelling that she wanted my name and the name of my supervisor. Both of which I gladly provided for her.

A few hours later, I received a call at the squad building from the medical director of the nursing facility. He wanted to know my side of the story. I told him the whole thing.

"Ah, yeah, it's easy to see why you would think that the patient was dead," the doctor said. "I'll have a word with the staff." Which he did. In fact, he called me again to say that there was a doctor in the room who did pronounce the patient. He also said that he had removed the parrot from her position of nursing supervisor for the way she acted toward me. Go Me! I'm putting together a course on Public Relations. It'll be huge!

I was called to another nursing home in Lawrenceville for a respiratory distress. The nurse was telling us the whole story on the way to the room. "He started to become a very grayish color, so I put him on oxygen."

We walked into the room and he was looking pretty pink to me. They had him sitting up in bed and on a nasal cannula. Because of a stroke he had, he could not communicate, so I started my assessment. Lungs sounded pretty clear, and the blood pressure was a little high. While I was doing my assessment, I kept getting distracted by this hissing sound. It was constant and driving me crazy. I couldn't take it anymore, so I started looking for the cause.

"He's looking much better now," the nurse said just as I found the source of the hissing. They had the nasal cannula, which is only supposed to be set between 2 and 6 liters per minute, set for 25 liters per minute. That's a bad thing. His nostrils were flared so much they looked like the entrance to the Holland Tunnel, and his eyes looked like they would pop out of his head any second now.

"Well, it must be your rigorous oxygen therapy!"

"Thank you," she said proudly. She nearly blows this guy's eyes out and she is proud of it. *Ma'am, I would sooner die than let you help me.*

I was called to transport a patient from a hospital to a nursing home in Jersey City. When I got to the floor, the nurses had big smiles on their faces. "Oh, are you here for Mary?"

"Yeah, I think so."

"All right!" Here's a lesson for those in transportation: it is never a good thing when the nurses are happy about a patient leaving.

My partner started to do the paperwork, and I decided to go see what we would need for the patient. As I walked down the hall, I heard a stereo blasting "Sugar Pie Honey Bunch." I like that song—or should I say I *liked* that song—so I started singing along with it. I rounded the corner into the patient's room and saw a sight that would forever make me hate that song.

There she was, this 90-pound seventy-three-year-old lady standing on her bed, singing at the top of her lungs, dancing, and twirling her dirty diaper around her head, naked as a jaybird. And if that wasn't bad enough, she throws the diaper toward me like a stripper throws her G-string into the crowd.

"Excuse me, nurse!" I said as I backed away from the room in horror. "I don't think she's ready to go yet."

"Why?" the nurse called down and beginning to crack up with laughter. "Is she stripping again?"

"Again? You mean she does this often?"

"Sure, all the time. I'll go change her now," she said as she walked down the hall laughing at me.

"Do you think you could maybe staple her clothes to her or something?" Then I called our dispatcher on the radio. "580 to Dispatch. This patient on 8C isn't going to be ready for another couple of minutes."

"Why not?"

"I'll call you on the phone and tell you."

"No, just tell me now."

"Because she isn't through doing her striptease yet," I fired back.

A long pause, and then, "I see. Maybe you should call me

on the phone and explain this." So I did, and we got a good laugh out of it. But for the rest of the day, everyone was singing "Sugar Pie Honey Bunch" when I walked by.

I was called to the same floor at that hospital a few weeks later for another transport. I had almost completely blocked that tragic incident out of my head. Fortunately for me, the nurses on that floor hadn't forgotten about it and so kindly reminded me of it. "If you liked Mary, you'll love Lorraine," the head nurse said. "Don't worry, she can't take her clothes off. But be careful, she might bite." She said it almost jokingly, so I didn't think anything of it.

I walked into the room, and I saw the look on the roommate's face. It was a mix of terror and relief that we were there. That was all I needed to see to know that this would be interesting. The patient was restrained to the bed with a mesh restraint vest. Her hair was sticking straight out. Her eyes looked sunken into her head, and they seemed unnaturally large. She had a snarl on her face that exposed her rotten teeth like Linda Blair in *The Exorcist*.

When we entered the room, she tried to struggle out of the restraints as if trying to get at us. Then she started screaming unintelligible things at us. Every now and then she would say something that we could understand like, "Get away!" or, "I hate you!"

We tried to undo the restraints, but she made a move at my hand trying to bite me. Then she started hissing and screaming again. "Ahhh, errrr, God is false, God is false!" Those screams caught the attention of the nurses and the doctors. They were gathered around the doorway looking at us.

Thinking quickly, I walked over to the sink, ran my hands under the water, turned back to her and started sprinkling the water on the patient. "The power of Christ compels you," I chanted as I sprinkled the water. "The power of Christ compels you!"

Everyone in the room started to laugh until she bolted up in the bed and screamed at the top of her lungs, "Ahhhhh!" That made everyone take a step back. But my makeshift exorcism must have worked because she gave us no more problems for the rest of the trip.

My friend told me that he was called to a respiratory distress at a nursing home in Jersey City one morning. While he was tending to his patient, he noticed a horrendous smell. The patient in the next bed had defecated herself. That's not the nasty part. She then proceeded to spoon handfuls of diarrhea out of her diaper and lick it off her fingers, expressing her pleasure with gleeful moans and giggles.

"Nurse!" he said. "You better do something about her before she gets sick."

And like any highly motivated and dedicated employee would respond, "She not MY patient!"

I was dispatched for a nursing home call; I forget what exactly the problem was but that doesn't matter. When we arrived, there was no nurse to give us the information on why we were there. We stood outside of the room waiting for someone to help us because we couldn't figure out why we had been called. So after a couple of minutes trying to track down a nurse, I did the only other thing I could think of: I hit the nurse call button on the patient's bed. I hit it several times, in fact.

After a minute of buzzing, the nurse came into the room—she didn't even notice we were there—and started yelling, "What do you want now, Mrs. Smith?"

What does she want? Well, let's try quality, competent, and caring healthcare providers for starters.

I had to transport a lady from a psychiatric ER to a nursing home. The patient was sitting in a room waiting for us.

We were trying to get the paperwork and talk with the doctor when I looked over my shoulder and saw her trying to climb up onto the stretcher. "Ma'am, sit back down in your room."

"Okay." She sat down in the room, and we went about checking over the paperwork. I looked over my shoulder again and she was trying to climb back up onto the stretcher. "Ma'am, sit down."

"Okay." She sat back down again. Finally, when it was time to go, she didn't want to get up onto the stretcher.

"It's okay, ma'am, you can get up now." So after much prodding, she got onto the stretcher and we left for the nursing home.

We arrived at the nursing home and I began to talk to the nurses. "So, let me ask you something. We were dispatched for her last night because she was an EDP. Isn't everyone in this nursing home an EDP?"

"Well, yes, but she was hitting herself in the head with the telephone."

"Why was she doing that?" my partner asked.

"Simple," I said confidently, "she was upset with her long distance carrier. I'd hate to see what she does when she realizes she paid a lot for her muffler."

THE MATERNITY CALL

My partner is in the ER having some tests run on him. Everything looks good for him so far. He'll be back to work in no time. Speaking of being back to work in no time, the chief finds me another partner and I'm back on the job. We shake hands and head out to snatch back lives from Death's ravenous clutches. It's now time for me to grab a quick bite to eat before they give me another call. Although I'm hungry, it's hard to decide what to eat.

I'm parked right in front of the donut shop, knowing full well that I should take advantage of this opportunity, yet I stall. I can't decide what I want to eat. It's a costly mistake.

As I reach for the door to walk into the store, my dispatcher calls over the radio. "Unit 5, I need you to respond to 857 Clendenny Avenue, apartment 8, for the woman in labor. Water did not break yet." *So close, and yet so far!*

I drive uneventfully to the location. As I drive slowly down the block searching for house numbers, someone runs into the middle of the street waving his hands. I slam on the brakes just in time to avoid running over him.

"She's having a baby!" He screams frantically. "The baby's coming now!" He lets out an excited yell and runs back into the house. I give my partner a what-just-happened? look and get out of the ambulance.

I take the stair chair out of the back of the truck, as well as a baby delivery kit. *Just in case.* I walk up a few cracked concrete steps and into the house. I see two doors in front of me. On each door there is a number. One and two. I do some quick math. *Apartment 8 is on the* fourth *floor.*

Just then we hear yelling and screaming coming from up the stairs. There is a commotion; a group of people are moving around somewhere in the building. "Hurry up!" A hoarse voice yells to us. "She's having the baby, it's coming!"

The adrenaline starts pumping. *They must be making a commotion over something, right?* The one thing I have yet to do is deliver a baby, and I don't want to do it today. I sigh and begin mounting the staircase.

By the time I reach the third floor it has become all-too-clear that I am not in shape. My legs ache, I'm out of breath, and I have a metallic taste in the back of my mouth. I look at my partner, who's in no better shape, still making his way up from the second floor.

The commotion is getting louder. When I reach the fourth floor, I see a large group of people in the room. Seven or eight small children are running around the room. In the middle of the crowd I see a young girl lying on the couch. She is crying and moaning.

"The baby's coming!" they yell as we walk through the door.

"Ma'am, how far about are your contractions?" I ask between large gulping breaths.

"Five minutes." She answers back.

"Is this your first child?"

"Yes."

"And has your water broken?"

"No."

I made a mad dash up four flights of steps and she's not going to have the baby for another couple of hours!

We get the important information and have her situated on the stair chair before I am able to catch my breath. "Now, listen up," I instruct her. "Do not reach out for anything while we carry you downstairs."

"Carry me?" She answers with a confused tone. "Why not use the elevator?"

Elevator? Elevator? For a fleeting moment I want to find the man who I almost ran over and rip his lungs out through his mouth. But I guess that would be wrong. It sure would have been nice to know about the elevator *before* my lungs collapsed.

OB/GYN DISASTERS
AND OTHER GENITAL ODDITIES

Some of the most disgusting calls to deal with are gynecological emergencies and other injuries to people's genitals. That's probably because most people feel awkward about checking out other people's nether regions, especially when they are funky and disease ridden. In a perfect world, we wouldn't have to deal with that ... and I would have won the lottery and moved out of my parents house a long time ago. Thus, we must face nasty rotten vaginas and elephantitis of the testicles.

I can still vividly remember my first call as a paid EMT. I had gone down early to the first aid squad in Lawrenceville for my volunteer shift. I was approached by a very red-faced per diem holding a towel around her waist. "Dev, I sort of split my pants. Could you cover for me for the last two hours? I'll pay you the two hours up front."

I figured what the heck, what where the odds I would get a call? I took the money and went to get dinner. As usual, right as I sat down to eat, we got a call for a "bleeding."

Doing the usual compliment of cursing the patient out

for ruining my dinner, I put my sandwich in the fridge and hopped on the truck. We pulled up on the scene and I grabbed the jump bag off the ambulance.

I could smell the coppery stench of blood as I walked in the door. Not knowing what was causing the bleeding, I started to get worried thinking that someone was in trouble. I became even more worried when I looked at the bed as I passed through the hallway. The sheets were soaked with blood and there was a very large blood trail leading from the bed to the bathroom.

"Hello?" I said with a hint of concern in my voice. "Anyone home?"

"I'm in the bathroom."

"Are you okay?"

"No, I can't stop bleeding."

"What happened?" I asked as I walked into the bathroom. The scene I saw was something out of a slasher movie. Everywhere I looked, there was blood. The toilet seat was dripping with blood, the water inside was red, and the floor was one puddle of blood. There was blood on the walls. I swear there was even blood on the ceiling. And in the tub, naked (as if she would be any other way) was a two hundred and twenty-five-pound lady.

"Help me, it's my period!"

At that, I looked at my female partner, and said, "This is *all* yours."

As I walked out to the truck to get the stretcher, I could hear my partner inside yelling like a Marine drill sergeant. "Do you have any pads? Yes? Then slap two on and walk to the ambulance. What, you can't walk? Have you tried? No? I didn't think so, let's go. You made it into the bathroom okay, and besides, exercise is good for you!" The only thing missing was for my partner to call her a "dirtball" or "maggot." *Actually, come to think of it, she probably did and I just didn't hear her.*

My partner came out, walking the patient. She walked her right into the truck, where the patient collapsed the wrong way on the stretcher. "Devin, lift up her legs to stop the bleeding."

"What?" I said, almost in tears. "I don't want to touch her."

"Come on, it's just blood."

"That's not just blood coming out from that place!"

When female friends complain about their periods and say I don't "understand" . . .

A friend was dispatched to a call in Trenton for an unknown medical emergency. In the world of EMS, "unknown medical emergencies" generally equal fun because the dispatcher can't bring himself to go into details over the radio. When he arrived on scene he was met by a lady at the front door in her early thirties. She said she had a tick in her private areas. Yes, that's right, he was called for a bug in her cootchie. When he looked, he couldn't find any ticks but he had a hunch. He asked her to point to it and she did. Apparently she has the world's unhappiest sex life if she thought that her clitoris was a tick. That's not something you want to wait until you are thirty to discover.

I was called one night in Jersey City for an unknown medical emergency. When we walked in, we were met by a frantic grandmother. She was crying that her granddaughter was bleeding from her privates and that something must be seriously wrong.

"How badly is she bleeding?"

"Oh, very bad, very bad!"

"Does she have any abdominal pains?"

"Ah, yeah, very bad, very bad!"

"Where is she? We need to talk to her." The grandmother directed us to the patient who was in her bedroom. The twelve-year-old girl was sitting on the edge of the bed, clutching her stomach. "What's wrong?" I asked.

"I'm getting these cramps and I was bleeding a little, from down there."

"How much?"

"Not that much, but it didn't stop yet."

"Honey," my partner asked, "have you gotten your period yet?"

"I don't think so."

"Well, I think you just did."

We transported her to the hospital with her still frantic grandmother. We sat her down in the corner of the waiting room and went to talk to the triage nurse. I gave the report to the nurse who just looked at me and asked, "Are you serious? You brought her here because she is having her period?"

That has got to be traumatic for the young girl. Here she is, taking that important step toward womanhood, and grandma calls the ambulance thinking she's dying. More baffling is this: why would grandma think something is very wrong? Didn't she go through that herself, or with her three daughters? Or did she just call the ambulance for them too?

I was called into Trenton one night for a maternity. The report on the radio was that the girl was fifteen, and her water broke. We arrived on scene to find a large group of men outside the house. Inside, there was the patient and her grandmother waiting for us. Grandma was just so happy that her little fifteen-year-old was going to give birth. My mother would have killed me if I was a girl and got pregnant.

Seeing that her water did, in fact, break, we decided to get a move on. Not because we were afraid that she would give birth in the ambulance (this was her first pregnancy and would probably be in labor for a few hours), but because it really began to smell nasty after that.

"Miss, what's your name?" My partner asked. All she

would do was her breathing exercises. "What is your name?" My partner asked again, getting a little annoyed. She gave him a nasty look and continued to ignore him and concentrate on her breathing. "What is your name?" Again, just heavy breathing. "Okay, so your name is 'Whoof Hoof'? Is that hyphenated?" And trying to get some sort of response from her, "Is that tribal? How exactly do you spell that?"

"My name," she said very indignantly, "is Quadrayah."

"How do you spell that?"

Getting even more annoyed, as if we were supposed to know, "It's spelled Q-U-A-D-R-A-Y-A-H."

"Oh, I see," I chimed in, "you spell that the common way!" My partner was choking back the laughter, but she didn't find the humor in that.

"I want the father to come with me. I ain't leaving till the father comes with me."

And without even realizing my slip, I said, "Do you know who the father is?"

"WHAT?" she screamed.

"I said," catching myself, "do you know *where* the father is?"

"He's outside." she said. *There were half a dozen men outside, could she be a little more specific?*

"His name is Carlos."

So I popped my head out of the ambulance to summon the father. "Which one of you is Carlos?" I shit you not; every one of them looked at each other like they were afraid to admit to me who Carlos was. "Hey gang, this ain't a tough question. At least one of you is named Carlos, and I want to know who that is. I'll even narrow it down. One of you is Carlos and he is the father of the baby."

"That's me," one of them finally and reluctantly admitted. He had to be at least twenty-five.

"Alright, she wants you to come with us. Come on."

He looked at me, then looked at his boys, looked back at

me, and then walked down the street with his boys. "Hold on," he said to me.

"Bud, you don't seem to understand the situation here. Let me help you figure it out: She's pregnant, it's yours, you're coming with us, and we're leaving now. Say good bye to your boys and let's roll."

With a huff like a child that doesn't get what he wants, Carlos finally decided to come with us.

That, my friends, is a sure sign that child is going to grow up perfectly fine and perfectly normal. Nice strong family structure, caring father, what else could you ask for?

A friend was riding for a squad near the New Jersey shore when he received a call for an "entrapment" in the bathroom of a municipal building. When they arrived, they were informed that 'Tiny' (as the other workers called him) was stuck in the bathroom. They walked into the bathroom to find a six-foot five-inch, 375 pound man sitting on the toilet. His pants were around his ankles. "Sir, what's the problem?"

"My ass is stuck."

"What?"

"I said my ass is stuck. See, I never shit at home, I always do it when I'm working. That way I get paid for it. Anyway, I was reaching to wipe myself and one of my rolls of fat slid through the hole in the seat. That pinched me, and I kind of jumped. When I jumped, another roll slipped into the hole. Now I can't get my ass out."

Yes, folks, these things *do* happen!

An ambulance was dispatched to a shopping center in a town that will remain anonymous, for an impalement in the sporting goods department of a major department store.

The ambulance and fire company arrived to find a rather large lady sitting on the ground screaming in pain. A bicycle was between her legs. When one of the firefighters went to move the bike, it wouldn't budge and she screamed ever louder. "I think it's stuck!" she screamed.

Sure enough, she had been trying out a bike when the seat broke and she was impaled through her butt. But this lady's luck didn't stop there. A genius on the fire department decided that they were going to use the cutting torch to cut some of the bike away. The only problem was that the metals in the bike conducted the heat to the point that she was getting burned in her rectum. *Rectum? Damn near killed 'em!*

Sometimes, a quick, funny comment can be just the thing that makes an otherwise painful moment bearable.

An ambulance in Lawrence was dispatched to a bleeding. When they arrived, they found a young lady bleeding from her vagina. Realizing that it would probably be a lot neater if she caught the blood clots as they fell out, the crew chief decided to get a bucket.

The crew chief was a nurse in a Labor and Delivery Department of a local hospital, so when the patient said she was on birth control, denied being pregnant, said she was having a regular schedule of periods, the crew chief wasn't too suspicious of a pregnancy. *Either way*, she thought, *if it is a miscarriage, I can collect it easier in the bucket.*

The mother came back with a bucket, and they allowed the patient to pass some clots into the bucket. As the patient began to relieve herself, large clumps of blood started to come out too. Then, a really large clump fell out, and the patient was done. The crew chief took the bucket and examined the contents.

To her shock, the last, large clump began to move. It suddenly had tiny arms and legs. Then the crew chief, who *never* curses, turned to her partner and screamed, "Oh SHIT!"

At about the same time, an ALS crew was arriving on the scene. As they walked into the house, they were greeted by the patient's husband and mother. The mother looked up at the paramedics as they came in and asked, "I have some Valium for my nerves. Do you think I should take it?"

Not yet knowing what was going on, the paramedic said no. Then paramedic saw the ambulance crew chief coming in the room, doing CPR on a baby no bigger than the palm of her hand. The paramedic looked at the patient's mother and said, "On second thought, take one of those valiums . . . Better yet, take one for me, too."

I was dispatched for a bleeding at a senior citizen highrise. When I reached the room, the patient's wife directed me to the bathroom. There was a trail of blood leading from the bedroom to the bathroom, and a large puddle on the bed.

The man was sitting on the toilet, naked of course. "Sir, what's the problem?"

"He pulled his catheter out," his wife said.

"I have a boo-boo," the man said to me. He had a look on his face like a little boy who just scrapped his knee.

"Sir, you have a boo-boo that no man wants to have," I said in a serious tone. "Why did he remove his catheter?"

"The bag ripped and he yanked it out."

"That was completely unnecessary. Sir, are you feeling dizzy?"

"Yeah, but that's because I am trying to finish shitting."

"Well, take it easy, don't blow an O-ring, let us know when you're done." My partner instructed him. "Someone has to watch him, we'll shoot for it," he said to me. Guess who lost?

So there I am standing in this little bathroom, holding him from falling off the toilet, coaching him like a Lamaze instructor, with the smell of blood, urine, and feces all around me. Luckily, just as I was about to pass out, he said he was finished. My partner joined me in helping shift him over to the stair chair. And as we lifted him over, we found out he wasn't as finished as he thought. A clump fell out and narrowly missed my partner's boots. "Uh-oh, code brown! Code brown!" I said with glee as my partner nearly fainted in disgust. Then he looked at me deviously and started to laugh an evil laugh.

"What's that for?"

"'Cause, my young friend, you're driving. Driver's responsibility to clean up the truck and the stair chair, and he just went again."

A friend was telling me stories of his days as an EMT in the area of a university in New Jersey. One evening they were called for "an injury" to one of the off-campus fraternity houses.

When he arrived, he found a bunch of frantic, drunk frat brothers, some of them in their underwear, running around screaming that they had to help this guy. There was one doubled over in pain, holding an ice pack on his genitals, crying his eyes out.

He couldn't talk because he was crying so much. They moved the ice pack and saw his penis was swollen and turning purple. "What the hell is going on here?" he yelled. Then a drunken man came up to him, identified himself as the Pledgemaster, and began to tell the twisted, painful story:

"The whole point is to trust your brother," he began. "So we got the pledges drunk and made them strip down. [*That statement alone can only signify great things are a'coming!*] Then we tied one end of a string around their penis, and the other end around a brick. We blindfolded them, cut the string without them knowing it, and then told them to drop the brick. Only problem was that we got really drunk and forgot to cut his string."

Okay, folks, we're going to take a time out to analyze this one.

1. Stupid things like this are the reason I never joined a fraternity.

2. How drunk do you have to be to: (A) let someone tie anything around your penis, and (B) think up something like this?

SEX INJURIES

WARNING: this chapter contains graphic depictions of sexual actions and lewd behavior. If this sort of thing disgusts you, please skip ahead to the next chapter. But, now that I have your attention . . .

It never ceases to amaze me how people can mess up a simple task like sex. How hard is it to turn each other on, get it on, smoke a cigarette, and then fall asleep? Maybe I am a little naive, but if sex ever gets boring enough that I have to resort to trying some of the following, please shoot me.

Going through high school, we all heard stories of women placing weird objects in their vaginas. I remember hearing stories of girls placing frozen hot dogs into themselves, or smearing tuna fish over the area and having the cat lick it off. I even remember hearing a story of a guy whose dog bit him in the testicles because he had smeared peanut butter on his penis to have the dog lick it off. There's no way I could say those were true. *But I wish I could!* The following, however, are all true.

★   ★   ★

I was dispatched one night to a confirmed cardiac arrest. While en route, we were informed that the police were being dispatched because we might have to force entry into the patient's house. I started to wonder how it could be a confirmed cardiac arrest if no one could gain access to the patient.

When we arrived on scene, we did have to force entry. After prying open the front door, we searched the house until we came to a locked bedroom door. Once inside the room, we saw a rather large, naked man faced down on the bed. We heard a female voice crying for help but didn't see anyone. That is, of course, until I saw two sets of small arms and legs kicking from under the man.

We rolled him over and found him to be in cardiac arrest. The paramedics and myself began CPR on him while my partner checked to make sure the woman was okay.

"I don't understand what happened," she began to say. "One minute he's feeling frisky, the next he collapses on top of me."

"Does he have any medical problems or take any medicines?" my partner asked.

"Yeah, he takes some medicine for his heart and his blood pressure. He said he just started taking something new tonight but I don't know what it's for. I'll go get it." She left the room for a few minutes and came back with his medicines. "They are Lasix, Digoxin, and this is the new one, umm, Viagara. Have you ever heard of that before?"

For anyone out there that may be thinking of starting, check with your doctor before using Viagara, please! This guy didn't.

From the City of Brotherly Love, Philadelphia.

A medic unit was dispatched to a house for two unconscious people. When they arrived on scene they found a young male and female naked on the bed. They were unconscious with no palpable blood pressure. The crew searched the room for any sign of drugs or alcohol, but nothing could be found. The crew was able to stabilize the patients and get them to the hospital. The case seem to bother the police enough that they got the parents of the young man to consent to a search of the house to find any kind of clue as to what happened.

The police uncovered a few condom wrappers in the trash along with an empty tube of Nitroglycerin paste. For those who don't know, Nitroglycerin dilates the blood vessels and lowers the blood pressure. When the man regained consciousness, he admitted that he grabbed the tube from his father's room thinking it was lubricant.

Hoboken, New Jersey. An ambulance and a paramedic unit were dispatched one night for a "traumatic bleeding." When the crews arrived on scene they were greeted by a very attractive young lady in a naughty little Victoria's Secret outfit. She was covered in blood and was very anxious.

"Right this way, it's my boyfriend."

As they entered the bedroom, they found a young man doubled over in pain holding a blood-soaked towel over his genitals.

"Sir, what's wrong?" They tried to ask, but it was pretty obvious he wouldn't be able to answer due to his screaming.

"It's kind of embarrassing. We decided to try anal sex tonight for the first time. And see, he's not circumcised— well . . . actually, *now* he is."

Somehow his foreskin got caught on the way in and was ripped back halfway down the shaft of the penis. I guess that's a powerful argument in favor of circumcisions.

The hardest working woman in Jersey City:

An ambulance was dispatched to a street corner known to be a big prostitution area, for a rectal bleed. When they arrived, a ragged, thirty-five-year-old lady approached them.

"Ma'am, what's the problem?"

"Well, I just tried anal sex for the first time today and my ass is bleeding."

"Well, that usually happens."

"Wait," the driver said, "didn't I bring you in last week because you were pregnant?"

"Yeah, I had a C-section."

"And you are back out here already?"

"Yeah, I gotta make money somehow."

I guess most pimps don't allow time off for maternity leave.

This next story comes from Weehauken, New Jersey. Many EMTs have experienced something like this, but this was the first time I was told about it.

The ambulance and fire department were dispatched one night for a motor vehicle accident with entrapment. When they arrived, they found both occupants of the car in critical condition. The female passenger was unconscious and wedged under the dashboard. The male driver was bleeding profusely and slipping in and out of consciousness.

The victims were cut from the car and rushed to the hospital. The paramedic in one ambulance attempted to intubate the female passenger. He was having a lot of difficulty due to an object clogging the airway. He managed to pull a bloody, fleshy clump out of her mouth. "What the hell is that?" the EMT who was in the back the ambulance asked.

"What do you think it is? It's the driver's dick!"

For the folks following along at home who may not already know, road hummers are a very dangerous practice and should only be performed by trained professionals. In other words, guys, if you don't have the control of a porn star and the concentration of a chess player, don't try this on the open road.

An ambulance was dispatched for an accidental injury. The patient, a man, was found in the bedroom on the bed, in the fetal position, crying his eyes out. "My nuts are swollen."

"Sir, how did that happen?"

"I'm not sure." *Bullshit. The one thing a man knows everything about is his nuts.*

"Sir, were you engaged in any kind of rough sex act?" *Of course, why else would he be in this chapter?*

At that question, the man's girlfriend became very irate. "How dare you ask that? I am a lady."

Seeing that this conversation was going nowhere, they decided to transport the patient. Once inside the ambulance, the story predictably changed. "Um, well here's what happened. Me and my girl was getting it on. I guess I was getting her hot because she was going wild. She climbed on top and started riding me. Then she starts really bouncing on me. Then it happened. I got this horrible pain in my nuts. I looked down and it was all disgusting looking."

As it turns out, she managed to dislocated his testicle. *Some lady, eh?*

An ambulance was dispatched one night for a vaginal bleeding. When they arrived, the crew found a nineteen-year-old girl in her bedroom, crying, with blood coming from her vaginal area.

"Ma'am, what's the problem?"

"The bottle cut me?"

"What bottle?"

"Well," very reluctantly, "I was masturbating with that glass bottle over there. When I had an orgasm, I clamped down on the bottle and it broke inside of me."

And who says masturbation is harmless?

My partner Wendell was dispatched for an EDP. When he arrived, the police officers were standing in the doorway smiling. "We would have canceled you, but you just have to hear this."

"Okay," Wendell said putting the equipment down, "go

for it." Wendell looked in and saw three attractive women sitting on the bed, all in bathrobes. The one in the middle was crying hysterically.

"Well, first off, this is one fucked up pussy eating story! The two on the end convinced the one in the middle to join them in a lesbian threesome. [*Well, if I didn't have the complete attention of every man reading before that statement, I'm sure I do now.*] This would be her first lesbian experience. So they are getting into it, when her boyfriend comes home from work early to surprise her. She forgot he has keys, and he lets himself in. Now, normally, most men would either watch or try to join in. What does he do? He calls 911 because he thinks his girlfriend must have gone crazy."

An emergency room doctor once told me that he had a man come in who was complaining of severe abdominal cramps. The doctor listened to his bowel sounds only to hear a humming noise. X-rays showed a seven-inch vibrator in the man's rectum. His friends admitted that they had inserted the device into the man's rectum after he passed out at the bar because he was being an asshole to them. The vibrator was in and turned on for over fifteen hours. The ER and OR teams started placing bets on what type of batteries were in the vibrator. I now know to always buy Energizer. Maybe they should change the mascot from the bunny to a dildo.

A man came into the emergency room in Hackensack, New Jersey, complaining of having something stuck in his rectum. Sure enough, he had a dildo embedded in his unholiest of places. But unlike the previous story, he put it there himself. He said that he had put so much lubricant on it that when he was teasing himself in the rear, it slipped out of his hands and became lodged. He also said that it was "one of those that gets bigger when it gets wet." *Gee, I wasn't aware that there was THAT type.*

Anyway, now he can't get it out. After exhausting all possible options, the ER staff felt that their only choice was to yank the sucker out. As they were pulling it out, the man barely made a sound more that a few moans. As they literally tore the ass out of him, he hardly moved. He just sat there, bent over, with his head down letting out little grunts and moans. Finally the object was removed, and the patient seemed to spasm and let out a sigh of relief. That's when a nurse noticed he had been masturbating the whole time they were operating.

A friend of mine told me this story that happened in a northern New Jersey town. The fire department was dispatched for a motor vehicle accident with entrapment.

When the chief arrived on scene, he reported entrapment but no accident. A young man and woman were stuck in the back of a two-door car. Both were naked and still in an embrace. Both looked no older than seventeen.

"What's the problem, young man?" the chief asked.

"I'm stuck."

"I can see that. Are you hurt?"

"Kinda."

"Can you move?"

"No, I'm stuck in her."

"You're what?"

"I'm stuck and I can't get it out."

After cutting the roof off of a perfectly good vehicle, the firefighters saw that the guy was indeed stuck inside of the girl.

"What happened?" the chief asked.

"It was supposed to be our first time together. We're both virgins. And she just locked up on me."

"Does it hurt?"

"Yes. I can't feel the tip."

"Didn't you try foreplay?"

"What?"

"Never mind. Let's just get you to the hospital." The EMTs had to secure both patients to the same back board and take them to the hospital. After heavily lubricating the woman, they were able to slide the penis out. Both kids acted predictably: the girl was worried that the doctor's would tell her parents; the guy was worried that his penis wouldn't work anymore. Now we know where his priorities lie. *And at least they'll both always remember their first time.*

My friend, Mike, was dispatched to an apartment building in New Brunswick, New Jersey, for a fall victim. An ambulance arrived on location, and less than a minute later, they were screaming for paramedics.

So my friend pulled up on the ALS unit. He saw that the patient was lying near a chain link fence, next to a five-story building. The BLS were securing the patient to a long board and stated he was unconscious. The patient's head looked like it was caved in near the right eye.

"We don't know if he jumped off the building," an EMT said to Mike. "He smells like alcohol, so he could have fallen out of the window. Whatever happened, there's hair in the chain link fence, so he must have hit that on the way down."

"How were you guys called?"

"I believe his girlfriend found him this morning."

So Mike left his partner to start the treatment and he walked over to the girlfriend to interview her. She was a wreck. "What happened?"

"Well, he stopped by last night after drinking at the bar. He was drunk and knocking on my window."

"Wait, window? Which floor?"

"Oh, the third. Anyway, he was knocking on the window, but I wouldn't let him in. I told him I didn't want to see him when he was drunk because he does dumb things.

So I told him to go away. He started to climb down. I went back to sleep. I thought I heard a crash, but I didn't think to look. When I came out to go to school today, I tripped over him going out to my car."

"What time did he stop by?"

"About three."

Okay, gang, let's break this one down. The dispatch time was about 8:30 AM. The patient fell around 3:00 AM, she left him out there for over five hours. She knows he does dumb things when he is drunk, like climbing up to the third floor window. She doesn't let him in and make him use the stairs to get down; she makes the drunken guy climb down. Then she hears a crash and doesn't for a second think that could have been her drunken boyfriend. That's love if I ever saw it. Completely oblivious people like them are also the most likely to wonder why dumb things like this happen.

I was dispatched to "an injury" one night. A girl who looked very scared greeted me at the door. Her boyfriend was in the other room yelling every profanity in the book at her and threatening to kill her. She had been going down on him and misunderstood him when he said it might be interesting to have her use a little more teeth on the tip of his penis. AN ADVISORY TO THE READERS: "a little more teeth" never means you have to bite his penis, especially not draw blood like this young lady did.

Another friend was dispatched for a "genital bleeding." When they arrived, a young lady met them at the door. She had drying blood around her mouth, and she looked very angry. They followed her into the TV room, where a young man was in the fetal position on the couch crying his eyes out. The lady waved her arms, grabbed a cigarette, and left the room to smoke it.

"What's the problem, sir?"

"The bu-bu-bitch bu-bit me."

"She bit you there?"

"Yuh-yuh-yeah."

"Why did she do that?"

"I don't kn-know. She was gu-going down and on and ah-ah-asked her wu-what the score of the hockey game was."

It never ceases to amaze me that some people don't know *why* things happen. You don't ask her what the score of the hockey game is when she's going down on you. Not even if it's the final game of the Stanley Cup. And if it's *that* important, try to look at the score without her noticing.

An ambulance from Lawrenceville was dispatched into Trenton for a choking one night. When they knocked on the door, a nasty-looking lady answered the door: ratty T-shirt, missing teeth, out of control kinky hair.

"Who called for an ambulance?"

"That would be (cough) me (cough)."

"What's wrong?"

"Well, I was (cough) down there with my (cough) boy-friend."

"Down where?"

"I was down there (cough)."

"Down where?"

"You know, (cough) down there." She motioned to EMT's crotch as she spoke.

"Oh, you were down *there*. And he finished?"

"Yeah (cough)."

"While you were still down there?"

"Yeah."

"How long ago was that?"

"Two days."

"Two days? He came in your mouth two days ago and you are still choking on it? You have got to be kidding me. More importantly, you want us to take you to the hospital? Just get your stuff and meet us downstairs."

An ambulance was dispatched in Lawrenceville one Sunday morning for an injury. The patient was outside of a gas station, walking sort of funny, waiting for them. "What's the problem, sir?" the crew chief asked.

"Well, it's sort of embarrassing." *Again, for those not in the biz, 'sort of embarrassing' usually means REALLY embarrassing.* "I was at the [one of Lawrenceville's beautiful welfare shelters] last night. We were having an orgy. And I heard that you could enhance your sexual pleasure by, um well, placing a nail in my urethra. So I did, and I forgot to take it out. I thought it would just come out when I pissed. But it didn't. Now I'm afraid that it is stuck." *So many jokes, so little time.*

You know who I feel bad for in this situation? The EMT doing the assessment. She had to look. So she took a peek, and nothing was coming out of the still erect penis. "Sir, I can't see anything."

"Well, that's because it must have gone further in."

"Okay, I'll take your word for it. All right, I'm gonna check your blood pressure now."

"Fine, I know the drill," he said almost proudly. "I'm an EMT for [an area first aid squad]."

The crew chief told me that they hung around the hospital long enough to see the X-rays. Sure enough, there was a nail implanted in the young man's penis.

Okay, folks, let's analyze this situation, shall we?
1. Why?
2. If you are an EMT, shouldn't you know better?
3. Apparently these orgies are a regular event at this welfare motel. *How do they do it?* The dynamics of carrying out an orgy at this motel are mind-blowing. The rooms are about the size of a closet.
4. I'm so glad that people are having so much fun on our tax dollars.
5. *Why?*

I was dispatched to the same motel one evening for an accidental injury. I walked into the room to find a large man in his underwear sitting on the edge of his bed. His girlfriend was sitting on the other side of the bed in her underwear. He was complaining of pain in his knee. I was having a real hard time hearing what he was saying because of the noise from the TV. I couldn't exactly make out what was on the TV; it was just loud enough to drown out what the man was saying.

"Sir, do you mind if I turn this off?" I turned to turn the TV off and, "Oh my!" He had some of the nastiest porn playing in his VCR. "Well, I guess I know what you were doing when you got hurt."

"Yeah, I got my girl [*who looked no older than fifteen*], I got my scrimps, [*that's right, scrimps not shrimps*], I got my booze [*a cheap bottle of Thunderbird*] and I was about to get my swerve on. We was getting into it and we fell off the bed."

Nothing ruins your night faster than falling off the bed, nearly breaking your knee, and having the ambulance and police find you doing an underage girl with alcohol in the room.

My friend was called for an impalement in a housing project in Jersey City one night. When he arrived he saw a young man in his twenties, with his leg impaled on the spoke of the fence around the building.

As the police emergency service unit was cutting the fence so they could move the patient, a large angry man came running out of the building. "You son-of-a-bitch, I'm gonna break your neck!" He was waving a baseball bat in his hands and was quickly subdued by the police.

The story came out in the ambulance: the young man was 27 years old. He was having sex with the angry man's daughter, who was only 15 years old. The parents came home while they were in the middle of getting freaky. Thinking quickly, the boyfriend got up and ran for the window. The only window that didn't have bars on it was the bathroom window. It was just big enough for him to squeeze through, but not big enough to see the fence below. He only became aware of it when he leapt from the second floor window onto the fence.

Another advisory to the readers out there, the man died because of his fetish. So please, if you do not want to die, or have people like me laugh at your misfortune, *do not* try this at home. *Or anywhere for that matter.*

Sean was also dispatched one night while doing his paramedic training time in Greenwich Village to an impalement. When he arrived he saw half of the emergency services in lower Manhattan outside of this apartment building. The police emergency services units were pulling the cutting torch off the truck; the fire department was setting up the Jaws of Life. No one knew what was going on. As they approached the house, a man came running out screaming, "Somebody do something, he's dying! Save him!"

"What's wrong, sir?"

"He's upstairs. I don't want to talk about it." Just a lesson here for those who may not know it yet: when someone tells you they don't want to talk about it, you're in for a treat.

As they ran up the stairs, another man came down the stairs. He appeared very calm and nonchalant in his silk pajamas and smoking jacket. "You must be here for me."

"Well, what's wrong?"

"I don't want to talk about it." Now if two people say they don't want to talk about it, you're in for a *real* treat.

"Sir, you must tell us what's going on."

"If you MUST know, I have an eggplant impaled in my asshole! Are you happy now?"

Without missing a beat, my brother fired back, "Are *you?*" Then, with much reluctance he said, "Sir, I know that in years to come I will regret asking you this, but can I see?" Sure enough, when he dropped his pants, he had an eggplant stem coming out of his anus.

Couple of things *very* wrong with this situation:

1. Why would one want to perform this sort of act with an eggplant? Pickles, perhaps. Cucumbers—why not? Hell, I'll even go as far as to permit the use of a banana if that's what floats your boat. But why an eggplant? Have you ever seen a ripe eggplant? It's pretty damn intimidating!

2. How does one get the *wide end* in first?

Now that I think about this, I truly don't need to know the answers to these questions. I firmly believe that I will be much better off in life if I am left in the dark about certain things.

RESPIRATORY DISTRESS

Finally, after three hours of trying to find the time, I now have a chance to eat my breakfast. Since we were delayed so long, the bagel shop downtown is now open. I order my ham, egg, and cheese sandwich (yeah, I know, not the breakfast of champions) and begin eating. Because I fear being interrupted, I eat so fast that I can't enjoy it. That's one of the downsides of this job. Anyway, it's better that I did inhale my food quickly.

"Number 5," the dispatcher calls, "I need you to respond to 338 7th Street, on the number two floor, for the party in respiratory distress. I have no ALS for you at this time."

I pull into traffic and start heading for 7th Street. The tail end of rush hour traffic has turned Grove Street into an ambulance slalom course. Cars seem to be stopping or double parked at such intervals that I barely squeeze by. I masterfully balance driving the obstacle course with one hand while downing my chocolate milk with the other. Every so often I have to hit the brakes to avoid hitting children that are crossing in the middle of the street.

I turn onto 7th Street and see a fire engine pulling up in

front of a house. Anytime someone calls with a life-threatening emergency in this city, the fire department responds to provide help to the ambulance. I pull in behind the fire truck and watch as the firefighters get off the truck carrying their defibrillator and oxygen.

We follow the firefighters up the stairs. I'm carrying the stair chair and our defibrillator; my partner has our oxygen. I hear a commotion coming from the second floor. People are yelling at each other and running around. I knock on the door and a young man answers it.

He looks at us questioningly for a moment. "Eh, you called for an ambulance?" I ask him. Without saying a word, he walks away from the doorway and sits back in front of the TV, allowing us in. "Which room?" I look at him, and he looks back but says nothing.

The sound of my voice attracts the attention of the other people in the apartment. Three middle-aged women come out from a bedroom and wave for us. "What's the problem?" I ask as I make my way through the cluttered hallway.

"What took y'all so long? Hurry! She can't breathe. She's having an asthma attack."

"Does she have asthma?"

"No."

"Then it's probably not an asthma attack."

There is another middle-aged lady sitting on the bed, tears in her eyes. "What's the matter, ma'am?"

Without pausing to take a breath she says, "I been having trouble breathing since yesterday and I can't breathe today and I can't stop coughing."

"Miss, if you can talk, you can breathe."

"No I can't!"

"Yes, you can." I take a listen to her lungs with my stethoscope and they sound normal, except for a little congestion. "I think you might have a bit of a cold. You're a little congested, but you're able to move good air."

"Don't tell me I can breathe—I can't breathe! And what do you know? You don't even look old enough to shave!" *It's always gotta come back to my age, doesn't it?* She stands up and paces around the room, flailing her arms.

"Look," I say trying to be diplomatic, "get your shoes and we'll take you to the hospital."

"Will you take me to Saint Francis?"

"Sure, why not?"

"I can't walk."

"Have you tried?"

"No."

"Let's go!" I guide her by the arm and walk her downstairs without any problem.

"I'll follow you up in the car," her friend calls to her as we walk downstairs.

Follow her up? You live two frigging blocks away. Why didn't you just drive her?

PSYCHIATRIC EMERGENCIES

I walked into the lobby of a psychiatric institution with a patient. The security guard behind the desk had a wide grin on her face and was shaking her head. "You look awfully happy this morning," I remarked as I signed the patient in.

"That's because I just found Jesus."

"Congratulations, that's wonderful."

"Yeah, they just escorted him upstairs to his room."

Some say that nothing in life is guaranteed, but I disagree. Emotionally Disturbed Persons (EDPs) are guaranteed fun. Just like fingerprints, no two EDPs are the same. The calls can range from hilarious incidents to physical fights. I will jump on an EDP call in a second because every one makes for a good story, *and the only time you have to carry them is when they are restrained!*

My first EDP call happened in Lawrenceville when I'd just started volunteering. We were called to a doctor's office because the patient he was treating had suddenly become violent. I was the smallest person on my crew, my two partners were about six feet, five inches and 225 pounds each. So they told me to stay outside with the Reeves stretcher and to pass it in to the office when they called for it.

They went into the office with three equally big Lawrence Township Police officers. I sat outside in the lobby reading a *National Geographic* and listening to the fight that was going on in the room. I could hear them yelling and furniture breaking. Finally my partner Randy stuck his head out the door and told me to pass him the Reeves quickly. When the fight stopped and they had the patient restrained, they brought her out. She couldn't have been more than five feet, two inches and 100 pounds. Never would I underestimate EDPs.

Once we had a 300-pound naked Haitian woman holding her baby hostage. She could only understand French. Of course the police knew that I took three years of French and asked me to translate. The only problem was that I had forgotten just about everything I learned in school, except how to ask someone to go to bed with me and how to tell them I want to have sex with them on the staircase. So they wound up having to Mace the lady and subdue her that way, which, in a way, was good because I wasn't prepared to ask her to go to bed with me. Knowing my luck, she would have said yes.

One of our crews was called out for a pedestrian struck on US Route 1. When they arrived, they were informed that this particular gentleman had consumed enough heroin to kill a herd of wild elephants, but that didn't kill him like he'd planned. He slit his own wrists and throat. Since that didn't kill him like he'd planned, he decided to run and jump off the overpass onto Route 1 in hopes of getting hit by a car. Surprisingly, despite the blood bath in his apartment, there was barely a drop of blood in his car. He parked the car, got out, and then leapt off the overpass onto Route 1. He broke both legs and nearly landed on a car. He was almost run over by a truck, but the thoughtful driver swerved to avoid hitting him. So he made it out with just two broken legs and several moving violations.

I have to give the Lawrence Township Police credit, not just because I am friends with many of them, but because they know how to keep on their toes. One afternoon, the manager of a local motel called the police because he heard a woman crying and throwing things in her room. The police entered the room and began to interview the lady. Her eyes kept drifting toward her purse. The officer noticed her doing this and went over to check the bag. She dove for the bag and they kicked it away. What happens to fall out but a loaded handgun! Then she breaks down and tells them she is from Idaho. She was depressed, so she pulled out a map, closed her eyes, and pointed. The place she ended up pointing to was where she would drive to kill herself. Of course it had to be Lawrenceville. Can you imagine the Jersey Chamber of Commerce jumping on that one? *New Jersey, You, and Suicide: Perfect Together.*

One of my favorite EDPs in Jersey City was Rosie. You always found Rosie at the same intersection, complaining of hearing voices that told her to hurt herself or complaining that her back hurt. Sometimes the voices told her to hurt herself *and* that she was having back pain, sort of like a two-for-one deal.

One night I was in a weird mood, and we got called for Rosie. I figured I could at least have a little fun. She was complaining of hearing voices as usual. "What are the voices telling you to do right now?"

"Well, nothing right now, they only talk to me when I'm in my house."

"Rosie, why don't you move then?"

"I'm afraid that the house I move into will have voices."

"Let me give you a little real estate advice. If you ask the real estate agent, 'Does this house come with voices?' she has to answer you truthfully. It's the law!"

"Really? I didn't know that."

"What's your phone number?"

"I'm not allowed to have a phone."

I thought, *this ought to be good!* "Why not?"

"Because I hear voices when I pick up the phone."

"Is it usually after the phone rings that you hear these voices?"

"How did *you* know?"

"I don't know, lucky guess."

One night I was dispatched for an unknown medical emergency and pulled up in front of a housing project in Jersey City to find one of the city's tragic victims of fashion illiteracy. This gentleman had one penny loafer on his right foot and a bowling shoe on his left. (The bowling shoe was for the right foot but somehow he managed.) He had the black tube socks pulled up to his knees, a pair of silk pajama bottoms, and a faded Bob Marley T-shirt that barely fit over his considerable belly. His head was bald except for a few braids on either side. Each braid had plastic seashells or butterflies in it. The sight of him alone had me fighting back a smile.

"What's the problem tonight, sir?" *Like I had to ask.*

"I'm hearing voices that tell me to kill myself," he said in a voice that seemed much too weak considering his body.

"Did you try to kill yourself tonight?"

"No, but I have in the past. Six times, in fact." And without further prodding, "Once I tried to swallow some aspirin, but that didn't work." *Well, thank you, Captain Obvious! For a minute there you had me worried that it* did *work.* "Then I tried to overdose on heroin."

"What happened with that?"

"Well, I called you guys and you came and saved me." Now it was pretty obvious that his suicide attempts may be a cry for help and that I should try to be a little more serious. Unfortunately, the more he talked, the harder it got for me. "Then I tried to jump out of my window."

"But, sir, you live on the first floor."

"Yeah, I guess that's why it didn't work. Then I tried to jump in front of a car, but the car just swerved. After that I tried to slit my wrists and lay in a tub full of warm water. But I guess the water wasn't warm enough." *Okay, let's stop this tomfoolery right now, shall we?* I really felt like taking my boot off at this point and knocking a little reality into him. But right on cue he kept on coming. "Then I tried to hang myself on the shower rod."

"Sir, you do realize that you weigh over two hundred and fifty pounds?"

"Yeah, well that's probably why it broke."

Yes, friends and neighbors, that's probably why it broke indeed. I do realize that this is the most insensitive statement I will probably say in this book (if you can believe that), but does anyone else ever get the urge to teach a class called "Suicide: Doing it Right"?

I once heard a story that a man in Philadelphia tried to kill himself by locking himself in his garage and turning the car on. The police and EMS were able to save him with no problems. Why? Because he ran out of gas before he could kill himself. *Come ON!* If you are thinking of doing it that way, wouldn't having enough gas be the first thing you'd think of? *I guess there's no need to keep him on suicide watch at the hospital; he wouldn't be able to do it right anyway.*

Here's an ungrateful patient: a distraught man attempted to kill himself by shooting himself in the chest with a shotgun. He loaded it up, placed the butt-end in the toilet and pulled the trigger. It probably would have worked if he had loaded the gun with buckshot instead of birdshot. The buckshot would have blown a large hole in the man's chest, whereas the birdshot only produced multiple, less severe holes.

The ambulance arrived, bandaged him up, and took him to the hospital. The man survived. After he had recovered and was released, he wrote a nasty letter to the rescue squad that saved him complaining about being saved. You just can't please some people.

Another night, I was called for a non-violent EDP. Hopefully, the call is screened before you are dispatched so that you know ahead of time if the person is going to be violent. Well, even the best laid plans . . .

Luckily a police car pulled up about the same time as us. A lady in torn up clothes with chunks of her hair falling out came running up to us with a lighter in her hand. She was screaming, "Satan lives inside of me! Satan lives inside of me! I must burn him out! The voices are telling me to burn him out!" *Okay, sidebar, Your Honor . . . How come the voices never tell them to, I don't know, say umm, get a job perhaps, or maybe take a shower. You know, do some productive things.*

Somehow the officer convinced her to put down the lighter. She then proceeded to rip out more of her hair and throw it at me. "You're the white devil. You are Satan. Get away from me, Satan!" *You know something? I had my suspicions for quite a while. . . . I mean, you've never seen Satan and me in the same room together, have you?*

"Ma'am, I promise you I am not Satan. Come on, we'll go to the hospital and get you some help. There are people there you can talk to. We can get you a counselor, or perhaps an Exorcist if that's what you want." Well, that did it, that set her off. She stopped pulling out her hair long enough to attempt to rip my eyes out. With a blood curdling scream and a ton of froth issuing from her mouth, she took a dive at me. Fortunately for me, the brick wall with a badge that some call a police officer jumped in front of her and restrained her.

Maybe it's a family thing, but people seem to often mistake me or my brother Sean for Satan. Why? We're good Catholic boys. We were altar boys in grade school. I just don't understand it.

Sean was listening to the radio when he heard a unit get dispatched for a twenty-year-old female with asthma in apartment 1E of an apartment building a few blocks from where he was. Normally he doesn't jump other people's calls, except that now it was a twenty-year-old female in apartment 1E. To him that meant (A) a potentially good-looking young lady, (B) no real carrying because she's on the first floor of her apartment building, or (C) asthma is usually a legitimate emergency.

He couldn't have been more wrong on any of those.

When he arrived, he found out that "1" was the apartment number and "E" was the floor, and no elevator. So he would probably be carrying the patient down five floors.

They huffed the equipment up the stairs and knocked on the apartment. He got no answer the first time, so he knocked louder. A voice came from behind the door, "Who is it?"

"EMS, ambulance." There was no answer. So he knocked again.

The same male voice spoke from behind the door. "Who is it?"

"EMS, you called for an ambulance?" No sounds after that. So Sean's partner pushed him aside and pounded on the door.

The same voice spoke again. "Who is it?"

"It's Barry and Sean. Will you let us in?" So now the guy

decided that he wanted to let them in. He opened the door and they walked in.

The apartment looked trashed, furniture and broken objects were thrown around everywhere. The middle-aged man who let them in looked beaten up. A scared grandmother sat in the corner pointing a shaking finger towards the back of the apartment. Neither of them spoke English, and the crew didn't know that much Spanish. But Sean and his partner thought, *How bad can an asthma patient be?*

They walked down the hallway, Sean first, carrying the large jump bag and drug box. The hallway was cluttered with some boxes and a small table. As he tried to pass, Sean became wedged between the table and the wall.

Just as he was trying to free himself, he heard a scream from the backroom. "Aye-aye-aye! You the devil. I kill you!" A look of shear terror passed over Sean's face, and his life flashed before his eyes as he saw a lady who was four feet tall and four feet wide come charging down the hallway.

It's amazing the things that pass through your mind as you are about to be killed. Instead of thinking, *Wow, she's going to kill me,* he was thinking, *How does she fit through the hall?* Lucky for him, Barry wasn't thinking about that. He reached over, grabbed Sean by the collar, yelled, "Gotta go, gotta go!" and yanked Sean free.

Sean and Barry ran for the door. And just like in a horror movie, the door wouldn't open at first. The man had locked it after they came in. Sean turned to see the lady pushing her way through the obstacles in the hallway. She broke free just as Barry got the door open. Sean felt one hand grab the back of his shirt and another reach up between his legs to grab the handle of the door. Barry yanked him into the hallway and closed the door at the same time.

They collapsed on the floor in the hallway, huffing and laughing. The door opened up, and the bewildered face off the man who let them in popped out. He looked at them for a moment, then a hand sprung out, grabbed him by the face, and yanked him in. "I kill you! You the devil!" Without even waiting to see her, Barry yanked the door closed again. They got up and ran down the stairs.

"12V to Central," Sean called on the radio, "we're gonna wait for radio. If the people call back, we're waiting outside for the police; we didn't abandon them."

"12V, is everything okay?"

"Not really. Call them back and find out why exactly they called an ambulance."

After a few moments, the dispatcher called back. "12V, we have further information on your asthma patient. She's actually a violent EDP. Use caution."

"Well, thank you," Barry said, "but we became painfully aware of that when she came charging down the hall trying to kill us."

The police arrived a minute later, along with a couple of concerned ambulances. They walked upstairs with the police. When they knocked on the door, rather than go through the whole thing again, Barry said, "It's Barry and Sean again. Can we come in?"

The man opened the door and he let them in. The patient was in the corner screaming that Sean was the devil. The police asked, "What's the problem?"

"Aye-aye-aye! I am possessed!"

Barry, who had a mustache and pointed goatee, started making devil ears with his fingers and saying in a deep, demonic voice, "She is not possessed. I did not possess her . . . *yet!*" A police officer shifted so that he was in front of Barry, who still continued to taunt her.

Sean, meanwhile, came up with another idea. He reached into the drug box and pulled out a small tube of Albuterol. (Albuterol is a liquid that is pretty much water, used to treat asthma patients.) He popped the top off and sprinkled the liquid on the patient. "See, you're not possessed. That was holy water."

She looked at him, stunned for a moment. Then she started screaming that she was burning. "Alright," the sergeant said, "I've had enough fucking around." He grabbed her by the arm, another officer grabbed her other arm, and they dragged her down the hall.

"Aye-aye-aye! I need my shoes."

"No shoes for you!" Barry screamed in his demonic voice. "No shoes for the devil, no shoes for the devil!"

My friend Henry was dispatched to a man's house when the caller said he could not walk because he had "bugs on his feet."

When he arrived, Henry found the man, barefoot, without bugs on his stinky feet, crying and jumping around. "They're biting me, stop them, they're biting me!"

"Sir, what's wrong?"

"I got bugs on my feet and their biting me."

"Okay. Not to say that nothing is there, but I see nothing."

"But they're biting me."

"Of course they are. Are you ready to go to the hospital?"

"Yeah, but I can't walk."

"Why not?"

"Because they are biting me."

"Listen, sir, in order to carry you, my partner has to put his hands right near your feet. And I'm sure he's not going to appreciate getting whatever funky bug you got, so walk. They haven't eaten your feet off."

What? Was there a shortage on real emergencies that day?

When I first started in Jersey City, I saw their invalid coach service as a great way to earn easy money. I just had to drive a van around town and pick up people who could walk or were in a wheelchair and take them to and from their doctor's appointments. Most of the patients can walk, so I was just a glorified taxi.

The first and only shift I worked on the invalid coach service started off great. It was a Saturday morning and there was only one person on the schedule. I spent most of my day hanging out at Liberty State Park and enjoying the wonderful weather. My four-hour break was interrupted by the dispatcher who told me to head back to the emergency room and to take home a discharge.

I found a young woman in the ER waiting room with her one-year-old son. He was mentally retarded, and I couldn't help but be touched by the affection she showed for her child. (Yes that's right, I do have a soft side.) We started making small talk on the way out to the truck, and I thought, *I could get used to this coach stuff.*

Just as we were pulling out of the parking lot, the dispatcher asked me to turn around and pick up another discharge from the Psychiatric ER. A strange, ominous feeling came over me; I knew my great day was over.

I met the patient just outside of the locked entrance to the Psych ER. Her left eye was swollen, her nose looked broken, and her bottom lip was split in the middle. I didn't want to pry, and I certainly didn't want to get involved in some runaway conversation about Communist conspiracies or alien abductions, so I didn't say anything. I made sure to sit her in the back of the truck.

No sooner did I sit her next to the first patient than she started doing just what I feared she would: she started talking. Her voice was just as I imagined it would be: high pitched and slurred—she lacked her two top front teeth. "Ssso, how y'all doing today? Girlfrien, what happened to yo baby? I guess you sshouldn't na been ssmoking crack while youz was pregnant." I nearly shit myself with that comment. I could see the tears forming in the young mother's eyes.

"I'll have you know that my child was just premature and there was nothing I could do about it, you crack-ho skank bitch!" *Whoa, hold on, ladies. Return to your neutral corners.* I somehow managed to keep them from killing each other.

But she wouldn't stop at that. "You better take me home first because I'm an EDP and I'll wig out if you don't."

I lost my temper at that. "You will do no such thing! And I will drop her off first because she lives closer!" She seemed to get the hint that she was pissing me off, so she didn't say anything else until after we dropped the mother off. As soon as I started the truck up and pulled into traffic, I heard a seat belt unbuckle and material slide up the seat.

Now she was right behind me, and I could feel her hot breath down my neck. The stench of cigarettes and stale human sweat permeated from her body. *Oh God, in the name of all that is good and pure, please don't let her talk, please don't let her talk, PLEASE!* "Sso, I bet you was wondering why I was in the hospital, aren't you?"

She spoke, SHE SPOKE, that's it, God has forsaken me! "Actually, I wasn't."

"Well, you ssee," *Holy shit, is she still going on?* "I was smoking some crack with my boyfriend [*BIG surprise there!*] and he was trying to sshort me. I was taking ssome hits but it wunt doing nuthing for me. Sso you know what I did? I took the pipe that you smoke it through, and I jammed it into his head. And when the cops came, I took a swing at one of them and they wrestled me down the stairs. That's how come my face is busted up."

As anyone who has worked with me can tell you, I have this annoying tendency to pick the longest, most congested routes to travel. I don't mean to, but it just happens that way. At this time, I was driving down Route 440 during the height of the Saturday afternoon shopping/lunch traffic. And I was cursing myself every step of the way for thinking that it might have been a good idea to take this route.

"Yeah, I gotsta kick my crack habit." *What the hell kind of word is 'gotsta' anyway? Wait a minute, she's still talking. WHY? I will give anything for her to just shut up.* "I tried heroin a couple times to see if I could kick my crack habit [*there's a well thought out plan if I ever heard one*], but I needs a cute little white boy to cook it up for me." And as if saying that weren't degrading and nauseating enough, she accentuated it by running her fingers through my hair.

"Sso, you gotsta girlfriend, baby?"

At the time I didn't, but I'd rather be circumcised without anesthesia than endure anymore time with her. "Yes, yes I do."

"I was hoping maybe you and me could get together sometime."

"Absolutely not!"

"Why? Is it because I'm black?" *No, it's because you are a crazy, disgusting, probably disease ridden crack whore.* But of course she wouldn't let me come back with a witty and profound statement such as that. No, she just kept right on coming. "'Cause ya know, I'm part white. Yeah, my mother is part Indian and I gotsta straight hair, ya know what I'm saying?"

There is a another thing I find highly annoying about myself. It seems that when I think a question to myself, an EDP will always answer it. I thought to myself, *What the fuck is she talking about? She's got an Afro so big I'm amazed she fits through a door.* But she must have been reading my mind, because the second I thought that, she said, "Yeah, I gotsta straight hair on my pussy."

Oh! Please tell me I didn't hear that!

"Why the hell are you telling me this? That is truly more than I needed to know. We're almost home; please don't say anything else."

"I'm sorry, baby. Come, we can still be friends, right?"

"Ma'am, we never *were* friends."

She was quiet for all of about a minute after that. Then, "Sso, do you and your girlfriend do the nasty?"

"What? That's none of your business. Please just shut up!"

"Come on, baby, what's your phone number?"

"My number's 9-1-1. Now get the fuck out!" I stopped the truck about five blocks from her street and threw her out. I drove back to the dispatcher center and told the chief what happened, got laughed at by him, and finished out my day with no more problems.

When I got home that night, I got a call from work asking me if I wanted some overtime because someone was sick. Being the money-hungry overtime slut that I am, I said yes. As I sat up in the crew room waiting for my partner to come back and meet me, I decided to listen to my scanner. Just as I turned it on, I heard multiple units, included an ambulance, our tour chief, the police Emergency Service Unit, and several police cars dispatched to *her* house for a violent female EDP.

As soon as I heard the crew calling for four-point restraints, I knew I just had to go to the ER and see. I made it to the ER just as they were pulling in. She was in The Bag, a restraining device used by the Police ESU to restrain a violent patient. It's essentially a body bag with a whole cut out at the top where hopefully the head comes out. She was cursing and screaming until she saw me. "Hey, baby! Come here, ssugar!"

"You know her?" my chief asked.

"Kind of, she wants me to come over and do a little cooking for her." I left it at that. The look of bewilderment on my chief's face was priceless.

An interesting side note to that story: About a year later, I was called to the West District Police Station in Jersey City for a non-violent EDP. When I arrived, I saw a police officer standing by a quivering mass of man. This guy on the ground was crying his eyes out as the officer tried to talk to him.

"Come here," the officer said as he pulled me aside. "This gentleman is a very nice guy, down on his luck, having a really fucked up couple of days. Make sure he gets treated okay at the hospital, please."

"Yeah, sure. I'll see what I can do. What's the problem?"

"Well, brotherman here is truck driver. He works his ass off so that he can provide for his woman. She's a little bit of a nut, but he's crazy about her. Never sleeps around while he's on the road. Well, the other day he went for an insurance physical and got rejected. Why? Because he has AIDS. Then he goes home and breaks the news to his wife. That's when she breaks down and tells him she's been giving guys ten buck blow jobs down on Cornelison Ave and that everyone in the neighborhood knew and was laughing behind his back. Now he wants to kill her and himself."

"Shit, I don't blame him." I went back into the ambulance and asked for his identification. When I looked at the address and last name on the driver's license, it was *hers*. Small world.

I was called to transport a lady from the psychiatric floor of the hospital to another psychiatric care facility. This lady seemed okay enough at first. Her fashion sense was a little off, but I expected nothing less. She was wearing a powder blue Hawaiian shirt that had yellow stains under the armpits, bright pink corduroy pants, and fuzzy faded pink slippers. I'm usually okay until they start to talk, and this lady took the cake.

I'll call her Edith, because when she talked, her voice was shrill and whiny like Edith Bunker from *All in the Family*. "Oh, where are you guys taking me?"

"They're taking you to that place we discussed, Edith," the nurse said. "You'll like it there."

The moment she opened her mouth the connection to Edith Bunker struck me. I thought that I was the only one, and that I would be able to keep a straight face, until my partner JJ looked at me and started humming the theme from *All in the Family.*

JJ and I quickly played Paper-Rock-Scissors to decide who would be in the back with her. Guess who lost.

So I'm in the back with her, and she keeps rambling on, "Is this a nice place? I don't want to get raped there. Will I get raped there?" That wasn't so bad, but every time she said something else, JJ would chime in from the front with the theme song. *Play the way Glenn Miller played . . .*

"I don't want to get raped there. Because, when I put on my makeup, I'm a real looker." *Didn't need no welfare state . . .* "And you should see me. You'd want me!" *Everybody pulled his weight . . .* "So is this a nice place?" *Those were the days!*

A few days after we had dropped her off at this facility, we had to transport another patient there. He was supposed to be like Hannibal Lecter out of *Silence of the Lambs.* Our supervisor warned us, "Don't talk to him, don't get near him, make sure there are no sharp objects in his reach! Never turn your back on him. He tried to set fire to the pysch ward, and then he held some doctors at knifepoint. He'll be handcuffed and sedated, but if he gets loose, for God's sake, just jump and give up the ambulance. It's a shitty rig anyway." *Lovely!*

We managed to transport him without any problems. When we arrived at the facility, there was Edith like a welcoming committee. She was sitting on the front steps with two more ladies on her right. There was a lot of talking going on, as all the patients were allowed out at this time for a cigarette. Well, as usual, the conversations ceased at the right moment, just as Edith yelled at the girl next to her, "No, we can't do that! All it would take is one person to find out. Then everyone would be talking about us." Everyone looked at her for a moment, then went back to talking. Then the girl next to her threw up, looked around, got up and walked across the parking lot. Edith looked around, oblivious to what was going on, and said loudly, "I think someone must have thrown up because it smells and I don't think it was me."

JJ and I looked at each other and burst out into song, *Those were the days.*

We brought our patient upstairs and began the difficult task of wrestling him over onto the bed and restraining him. When that was complete, we turned to walk out into the hallway. Who to my surprise should I see but Edith climbing onto our stretcher. "I've had enough of this place. You brought me here, now bring me home!"

The doctor looked at me, gestured towards Edith, and asked, "You did this to us?" I looked at him apologetically and nodded. He looked at me and jokingly said (or at least I hope it was jokingly) "You bastards!" *Those were the days!*

The first EDP call I went on in Jersey City was for one of our regulars. We were actually called for someone with difficulty breathing. Of course, not knowing who she was, I was in for a real treat, and my partner so thoughtfully neglected to tell me anything beforehand about this lady.

When we arrived, I saw a lady in ragged jeans, a torn down-feather jacket, and laceless shoes standing by a pay phone waving us down. "What's the matter, ma'am?" I asked her.

"I'm having trouble breathing."

I then switched into my by-the-book mode. I immediately called on the radio for paramedics without asking her anything further, like the good EMT I was. Then I put her on oxygen, and listened to her breath sounds.

"I'll bet you a soda they're clear," my partner said with a grin.

"Yeah, they are. Good guess."

"Not a good guess, just good memory. When did the trouble breathing start tonight?"

"Right after they raped me."

Oh my gosh, I thought. *Someone raped her. Maybe I should call for the cops now.*

"Right after who raped you, ma'am?" my partner said with a wide grin and nodding his head in that yeah-yeah way we talk to someone who we think is lying.

"The aliens!" she said matter-of-factly.

"Aliens?" I said, not believing my ears. "Like . . . space aliens?"

"Yeah, Dev," my partner said, "she ain't talking about the ones from Mexico."

So rather red-faced, I walked her to the ambulance. "309 to Dispatch," I called sheepishly on the radio. "Cancel the paramedics, we'll be taking one to the [a city hospital] complaining of alien invasion."

Apparently, she isn't the only one in Jersey City who has been attacked by aliens. An ambulance was dispatched for an EDP on the corner of Tonnele and Broadway. This is important because that seems to be a magnet for EDPs and alien activity. *Maybe when the Martians visit Earth, that's where they land, or is it that they love to dine at the Finger Lickin' Chickin' place on the corner?*

Anyway, the EMTs arrived on scene to find a very agitated man standing outside by a phone booth. He was looking over his shoulders constantly, startled by every noise. "What's the problem, sir?"

"You need to take me to Christ Hospital. Hurry, there's no time!"

"Well, why isn't there time?"

"Because they're coming!"

"Who?"

"The aliens."

"Okay. And how do you know they are coming?"

"Because I have seen them walking around the streets. Here," handing the EMTs a piece of paper, "they look like this." On the piece of paper was just several streaks of color, with no discernible shape.

"Come to think of it, you know you're right," one of the EMTs said sarcastically, "I have seen them."

"Yeah, you see! So now you have to take me to Christ Hospital!"

"Well, why Christ?"

"Because when they lock you in that quiet room, only the nurses can open the door. So the aliens can't open the door. Plus, there's a lot of concrete and steel in the hospital's walls, so they can't beam me out!"

Attention readers: Be on the look out for floating swirls of color. If you see them, check yourself into the nearest hospital as soon as possible!

"Respond to the intersection of Summit and Magnolia," said the dispatcher, "for the man taking his clothes off in the intersection, possibly waving at cars as he does so." Yes, that's right, a man removing his clothes in the middle of the street. Maybe I should mention that this was in January and it was starting to flurry.

My first thought was that this had to be a false story. *What? Someone call in a phony call to 911? No, that never happens.* My partner felt the same way, too. Boy, were we in for a shock when we pulled up to see a three hundred-pound man in the middle of the street, in the buff, directing traffic! And doing a pretty good job, too, if you ask me. Can we guess what he was using to wave cars on? His . . . hands, *but I like the way you think.*

When he saw the ambulance pull up, he ran off down the street. He moved quite well for a naked fat man in the snow, I'll give him that. "Should we go after him?" my partner asked.

"Well, if we catch him, do you really want to handle him?"

"Good point! I'm sure the police will find him later. After all, how easy is it for a man to run naked in this city without getting noticed?"

"307 to Dispatch. We'll thankfully be back with no patient."

Yes, reader, "There are many moons in the naked city."

Can somebody answer this for me? Why is it that only people above the two hundred and fifty pound mark get those voices that say to take their clothes off in public? I just don't understand it. I just wish for once a Playboy Bunny might lose her mind and get naked and direct traffic while I'm working, just once!

I sometimes wonder how a dispatcher judges who is an EDP. Sometimes, I imagine that it is pretty easy. ("There are aliens in my TV set.") But other times . . .

I was dispatched one night for a female EDP. The dispatcher told me that she was hiding in her car, inside of a parking lot, behind a building. When we arrived, we found that the car was parked on the side of the road, and a woman was in the front seat. She saw us and got out to talk.

"What's wrong?" I asked.

"I'm being followed—for the last couple blocks."

"By whom?"

"By a man in a white car. See, here's his license plate."

"Okay. But you're not crazy, right?" Oh, come on, like you wouldn't have asked?

"No, I'm not crazy. He started following me at the State Highway, and he's been following me for the last couple of blocks."

"Why did you pull over here?"

"Because it's not safe to go home. What if he attacks me there?"

"Good point. But why didn't you just stop in the parking lot of the Dunkin Donuts where there are people around and call the police there?"

"I don't know."

Well, now we have gotten to the root cause of the situation: She's not crazy, but she has no common sense. While I agree she needs help, we certainly can't do anything for her. As far as I know, you can't rehabilitate someone's common sense once they have lost it. It's sad, I know, but we must all live with this fact.

I was dispatched to a Dunkin Donuts patient who called because he needed a shower.

When we arrived, a disheveled and dirty man stood in the middle of the parking lot. He was yelling something at a clean, well-dressed man near him.

"Sir, what's wrong?" I asked.

"You see," he began, "I am sick and I heard that a cold shower will help you get better."

"So you called 911?"

"Yeah, that's right. I need to go to the hospital so maybe they can give me a shower and help me feel better."

"In what way are you sick?" my partner asked.

"I was throwing up before, but I must have thrown up everything because I'm not throwing up anymore."

"When did you last throw up?"

"Two days ago."

"And you are still sick?"

"Yeah, he'll tell you," he said motioning to the well-dressed man.

"Hey, I don't even know who he is," the bewildered man said.

"All right," I said, "I don't have the patience to debate this. What hospital?"

We got in the truck, and I called en route ("305 to Dispatch, we'll be en route to the hospital for the wash down.") and I went to the hospital without using the lights or sirens. Five minutes into the ride, I heard the patient say something about making a 'scab sandwich,' and then my partner climbed up front.

"Hey, Dev," Wendell said, "let's make this a Priority 2 transport [with lights and sirens]. It's an olfactory emergency."

Just as he said that, I began to smell just how badly the patient stank. *At least he wasn't lying; he really did need a shower.*

We got him to the hospital without passing out and brought him in to the triage nurse. We explained the situation to the nurse, and he turned to patient. "What do you want?"

"I need a room. If you don't have any rooms, I'll leave. I'll have them take me somewhere else."

"The hell you will!" I said.

"Sir," the nurse said, "do you need a bed?"

"No, I don't need a bed. I can't leave with it. I need a room." *Wow, that's really a mind-boggling statement.* "They know me here . . . I got psych problems." Hold on, *him?* No. I won't believe it!

After five minutes of frustrating but amusing discussion, my partner and I left. What followed was an hour of ragging on this guy. But, if you think that's mean, we got our punishment.

Not much later, we were dispatched to right around the corner from the same hospital we dropped him off at for an unknown medical problem. It was him again. He had walked out of the hospital and called 911 from around the corner.

"What the hell do you want now?" my partner yelled.

"I want you to take me to the another hospital. They wouldn't help me here."

"What do you mean they wouldn't help you here?"

"They wouldn't give me a room."

"What do you think this is, a hotel?" I said.

"I need a bed so I can get some rest."

"If they don't think you need a bed, you probably don't. And if they don't help you at the hospital we take you to, are you going to call us to take you to a different one?"

"Yeah, probably. That's what you are here for."

"Hell no!" I yelled at him. "What does that say?" I pointed at the sign that says EMERGENCY DIAL 911 on the back of the truck. "That says *emergency*, and you needing a shower or a bed to sleep in is not an emergency. So I will take you to the hospital now, but so help me God, if I see you again tonight calling for an ambulance, I will call the police and have you arrested for abusing the system."

"Good," he said, "then I'll have you arrested."

"For what? You called me, and I took you to the hospital. I can yell at you for wasting my time if I want to, so long as I help you."

What I can't understand is this: This guy calls me because he needs a shower; yet I had someone who took the bus to the hospital after being stabbed in the chest. Why aren't people able to make that distinction of what is and isn't an emergency?

You know, there are times when I think of my calls like the wreck of the Hindenberg, that huge airship that crashed in New Jersey in the '20s with the radio announcer screaming, "Oh, the humanity! Oh, this is terrible! In all my years as a broadcaster, I have never seen anything like this!

I was called to an apartment for a violent EDP. As we approached the scene, we saw a man doing the ambulance dance on the side of the road. The police arrived at the same time as us, and the dancer said that there was a man in the apartment upstairs who was going crazy and breaking things. He also said that the man's mother was there and was possibly in danger.

We walked upstairs to find the patient standing in the kitchen, amidst a chaotic mess of broken furniture and other things. He was calm, smoking a cigarette, wondering why we were there. The police kept him busy while we checked on his mother. Satisfied that she was unharmed, we turned our attention back on the patient.

"Sir, what's wrong?"

"Well, I was in the shower, then they started pissing on me."

"Who?"

"Them! The little men. You don't see them? Of course not. They can make themselves microscopic when they snap their fingers. They jumped out of the shower and started to attack me."

"How 'bout we go to the hospital and get you checked out? Make sure those little bastards didn't hurt you."

The patient agreed and started to head for the door. Then he stopped, turned and said, "They're not coming, are they?"

"Who, the little men?" I asked. "Not unless they want to. But the rules say that only one can come and he has to sit up front with my partner."

"No, I don't want them to come with me. Can you make sure they aren't hiding in the ambulance?"

One of the cops laughed and shook his head, then walked over to the ambulance. "Okay, any little men better come on out right now!" Then he turned back to us and said confidently, "There are no little men in here."

We loaded the patient into the ambulance and set off for the hospital. Halfway to the hospital, the patient, who had been quiet all along, jumped out of the seat wiping his head. "What the fuck was that?" he yelled, quite panicked.

I looked up and saw that he was sitting under the hand wash dispenser. "Sir, that's just soap."

"No it ain't, that's one of them. He's pissing on me again." He became very red in the face and looked at the dispenser. "I know you are in there, motherfucker! Fuck you, you bastard! I'll kick your fucking ass, motherfucker!" He was giving the dispenser the middle finger and making a cross with his index fingers. "I'm on to you, you motherfucker!"

Hearing the commotion, my partner pulled over. The

police behind us jumped out of their truck thinking something was wrong. "What's going on?" one of the officers said. Hearing the patient yell that there was a little man inside of the soap dispenser, he smiled, then started yelling wildly for everyone to get out of the truck. Then, he drew his nightstick, climbed in the back, and started slamming cabinets. Finally, he yelled, "I told you to get out, now get out and stay out!"

That satisfied the patient, and he gave us no problem for the rest of the trip. I walked into the ER and started to give the report to the doctor. I said that we had an EDP and the patient said little men who can make themselves microscopic jumped him in the shower. Apparently the doctor wasn't listening to what I said because he asked, "So who did you bring in, the EDP or the person that was attacked?"

"You weren't listening, were you? The patient we brought in said that microscopic men attacked him in the shower."

After a brief pause, the doctor looked at me and said, "I hate you. Why did you bring him here?"

Walking back out to the truck in a very weird mood, I picked up my drink on the dashboard, drank a little, then spit it out in my partner's direction. "Damn it!"

"What?"

"That bastard pissed in my drink!"

"Who?"

"The little man in the soap dispenser." We both laughed, then I picked up the radio. "310 to Dispatch, we're gonna need some time to decontaminate our ambulance."

"What's the problem?"

"Apparently I have a little man that can make himself microscopic hiding inside of my hand wash dispenser."

After a drawn out pause, "Right. Telephone the desk immediately and explain this."

I was dispatched for an EDP one evening at a 'premier' motel in Jersey City. When we arrived, the mobile crisis team was on scene. They did not go in until we got there because the patient had a history of being aggressive.

We walked inside, and the patient was lying in the bed watching TV. "What are you guys doing here?" she asked quite surprised.

"We're here to take you to the hospital," the crisis workers said.

"But I don't want to go." Then conversation went back and forth for several minutes in something of a "you're going"/"no, I'm not" manner between the patient and the team.

Seeing a large bottle of rum and several empty beer bottles on the nightstand, I asked, "Have you been drinking today?"

"No, I quit that." She said it with determination, like she had been sober for several years.

"Really?" I asked. "When?"

"This morning." *Wow, a whole five or six hours. I'm impressed.*

The ESU truck showed up, and the police officers were more than helpful in getting her to go to the hospital. No beating around the bush. "The manager called and said you were getting violent. She doesn't want you here. You're going to the hospital!"

"But I'm not going. I don't want to be a radio. I ain't no one's radio! How can I enjoy myself, enjoy my body if she's always on it?" I looked and Wendell and he looked at me with an expression that screamed *The thought of anyone on her makes me ill!* "I don't wanna go to the hospital. They're gonna cover my eyes and make me a radio. I ain't no one's radio. Well, if I'm going to the hospital, I wanna bring my radio!" *Wow, is anyone else's head spinning after trying to keep up with that?*

As she was getting her things together to leave, the crisis team asked, "Have you been taking your medicine?"

"No. I don't want to take my medicine. It makes me lose my senses. It makes me blind. It makes me a radio. If I lose my sight I'm in the dark. And if I'm in the dark, I'll get horny."

With those profound words of wisdom I bit my tongue. I looked at my partner, and he was also holding back the laughter.

"Well, we have to go set up the stretcher!" he said to the team as he grabbed my arm and pushed me out the door. Once outside, we burst into tears with laughter. Sure, I feel bad laughing, but sometimes you just can't help it.

I was called to the Port Authority Police Desk at Journal Square, Jersey City, one afternoon for a non-violent EDP. We found the patient in the holding cell. I had a bad feeling because all of the officers were trying hard not to laugh.

"What's the problem, sir?"

"Ain't no problem. I just needed a Band-Aid or sumthin."

"Why?"

"Cuz I cut my toenails and they started bleeding."

Sure enough, his toes were bleeding at the tips. So I figured what the heck, I'll go in and clean him up. "Whew! What the hell is that smell?" There was a stench so bad in the cell that I began to dry heave. At that, all of the officers burst out laughing.

"He wasn't feeling clean," said the desk sergeant while he wiped the tears out of his eyes. "So he decided to freshen himself up for you. After we put him in the cell, we came back later to find him washing himself with the toilet water."

Breathing through my mouth, I managed to stay in the cell long enough to clean the blood off his toes. He had ripped out all of his toenails. *This man has to be crazy. How can you rip out your toenails and not be crying like a bitch?* Sure, I can understand bathing yourself in dirty toilet water, that's not crazy! *Hell, a man's gotta be clean right?* But I draw the line at ripping your toenails out. *That's just insane!*

Of course, as soon as I thought that, he said, "Just because I hear voices that tell me to hurt myself doesn't make me crazy. I'm just mentally disturbed."

What? Excuse me, isn't that the definition of crazy?

But the best line I ever heard was . . .

When my old partner in Lawrence worked for Trenton EMS, he was dispatched to the Trenton Psychiatric Hospital for an eye injury. TPH is the place where most of New Jersey's craziest of crazies go, usually the criminally insane.

After going through the usual process of pat downs, surrendering all sharp objects and probably a body cavity search or two thrown in for shits and giggles, they were led down the hallway to the patient's cell block. Dodging flying objects, urine showers, and a couple of unwholesome propositions, they found the patient's cell.

Inside, the patient was standing there with a pencil in his hand. On the tip of the pencil was his eye, optic nerve still attached running back into the socket. The patient was laughing his ass off like a hyena.

"Well, sir," my friend said, "thanks for keeping an eye out for us." *What else could you say?*

I was called one night for a 10-2 in Jersey City. That means that another unit is in trouble, usually with a violent patient. It was right around the corner from the hospital that I had just dropped a patient off at, so I hauled ass out of the parking lot. We pulled up to see that another ambulance was already there helping the first, and we knew two more ambulances, a paramedic unit, and our tour chief would be on the way to help out. One fire engine was there, and another pulled up just as we did. For whatever reason, no police were there yet.

The call was on the fourth floor of a housing project, and we decided to not wait for the urine-soaked elevator and ran up the feces-ridden stairway. The captain of the engine company led the charge up the stairs with a yell like a Civil War general and we all followed him.

So we made it up the stairs, pushed our way past the crowd, and saw a pile of EMTs and firefighters on the ground. Underneath them was a young man violently thrashing about. "What's going on?" my partner asked.

"We came here for a seizure call, he comes to the door all nice and calm, then he starts pushing us around. We knock him to the ground, and he starts flopping around like a fish. We tried to restrain him, but nothings working, he's too damn strong for us. So we called for help."

"All right, let's everyone get up for a second," ordered one of the paramedics.

The patient had stopped flopping around and looked like he was about to go to sleep. "Sir, are you okay?" someone asked. Then, all of a sudden, he started thrashing about again, banging his head off the concrete floor.

Naturally, our first instinct was to hold him down so he couldn't hurt himself. Three people were on his legs, two on his arms, I sat on his chest, and a brave firefighter put his foot under his head. One leg came loose and kicked one EMT in the head, an arm came lose and punched me in my side, and the guy broke the firefighter's foot with his head. "That's it!" the paramedic screamed. "Everyone off of him. Let him bang his head into the ground. I don't give a fuck. Eventually he will stop."

So that was the plan: let him knock himself out. We didn't realize that my man was the Timex of EDPs. He took a licking and kept on ticking for about five minutes before we decided to jump on him again. Somehow we managed to tie his arms and legs together, and restrain him in a Reeves stretcher.

And of course, as we brought him outside, one patrol car came pulling up. "Oh, do you need us anymore?" I think he felt really bad when he saw us limping out, disheveled, and looking like we all went fifteen rounds with Tyson. I could have sworn I heard someone tell him to put down his Dunkin Donuts and go home.

A friend was dispatched for a suicidal jumper on the Hackensack River Bridge in Jersey City. They pulled up near the bridge just in time to watch him jump off into the icy, polluted river. They notified the Jersey City Police, who in turn notified New Jersey State Police marine unit. Dave pulled out his binoculars and sat back to watch the recovery.

"Oh no!" he yelled as he threw down the binoculars.

"What?" his partner asked.

"He made it! He's still alive. Now we have to listen to him complain the whole way to the hospital. Not to mention the fact that we have to get dirty to bring him to the ambulance. And the paperwork!"

They sat back and watched as the State Trooper in the boat came flying down the river. He reached out with one hand and yanked the jumper into the boat. Then he drove over to the shore and made him walk off the boat.

The crew started to secure him to a long board. As they put a collar on him, he started screaming like he was dying. "My ears, my ears!" So they gave a quick check to make sure that no fluid was draining out of ears, then continued to apply the collar. "My ears, my ears!" They checked again, and found the two little studs he had for earrings.

"Damn it, if you are going to scream about earrings, they better be more manly than these," Dave said.

After securing him to the board, they left the scene for the hospital. The man didn't say anything when they asked him questions, but then he got this goofy grin on his face and turned to Dave. "Was it a good jump?"

"That depends. Were you trying to kill yourself?"

"Yes."

"Then, no, it wasn't a good jump."

The man thought for a moment, then turned his head again with the same goofy grin. "Maybe next time."

On another occasion, I was dispatched to the Journal Square Port Authority Police desk for an EDP. She was sitting very quietly in the corner, wearing jeans and a muumuu that was so brightly colored I almost had to shield my eyes.

"Why is she wearing that?" my partner whispered.

It's like I said, fashion sense is the first thing to go when you turn crazy. Turning to her, I asked, "What's the problem?"

"See, the problem is this. I was released from the hospital two days ago and I was supposed to meet up with my mother here so she could take me home. Only, that bitch never showed up." *Please tell me you have not been waiting in this subway station for the last two days!* "I can't believe she did that to me. And I've been waiting here ever since." *Oh my god! She's been waiting in a subway station for her mother for two days. I really hope her mother is alive.*

"I don't want to sound insensitive, but are you sure she's coming? She's not . . ."

"Dead? Is that what you think? No, she ain't. Not until I get at her anyway."

"So, what's the problem today?" *As if waiting for her mother in a dingy subway for two days isn't crazy enough.*

"Well, I've been hearing voices." *Wow, there's a shocker!*

"Do they tell you to kill or hurt others or yourself?"

"No, I just hear people talking all around me."

"Ma'am, do you think that could have anything to do with the fact that you are in a crowded subway station?"

"Yeah, but guys are asking me for blow jobs." Well, now, that's not such a crazy thing.

And as we brought her out to the ambulance, something happened that made me think she wasn't all that crazy. Someone asked me for $20, then asked if she would give him a blowjob. So maybe she wasn't so crazy after all. Still, sometimes I feel that, the exception of my partner, I might very well be the only sane person I come into contact with at work.

There seems to be an unwritten rule that when a major catastrophe happens and you aren't assigned to it, something or someone crazy will happen to you. One night there was a major warehouse fire in Jersey City. The air was so humid that the smoke hung low to the ground. The major concern was whether or not the pesticides burning the building would hurt the people in the surrounding houses. So most of the city's EMS units were assigned to stand by at the fire, or to answer the many respiratory distress calls that the smoke caused.

I, on the other hand, was one of the unlucky ones that had to handle most of the city's other emergency calls. By the end of the night, I would have answered twenty-four calls in my twelve-hour shift. During the shift, I was called to a "violent, homicidal, suicidal EDP." And as if it needed to be said, they added, "Wait for the police." *Damn it, I wanted to get my ass beat by a violent, homicidal, suicidal nut. They never let me have any fun.* We sat outside of this house for twenty minutes waiting for the police. A patrol car drove past us, stopped in front of the house, and then kept driving.

When I asked the dispatcher what he wanted us to do now, he said, "You can leave. I guess if he decides to kill himself or someone else they'll call back. I have another one for you. The intersection of Palisades and Congress, see police, they have an attempted suicide."

Let's, for just a moment, break down that statement: Attempted suicide. Suicide is easy: to kill yourself. Attempted: to try. Usually 'attempted' signifies that you tried and failed.

When we pulled up, there were a dozen police cars blocking off the intersection. A huge crowd of people gathered around watching the two dozen police officers with their guns drawn, surrounding a young man who had a large carving knife and was carving himself up. He kept walking around, trying to get closer to the people in the crowd. Not only that, but he was making jokes as he did it, so at least he was a cheerful person when he was depressed.

"Do you have paramedics coming?" the sergeant asked me. "If he makes a threatening move at the crowd or an officer, we're gonna shoot him."

"Good idea. I'll call for them now." So I radioed for paramedics and was informed that none were available. Then the dispatcher asked me to call him from the payphone on the corner.

"What's going on with this patient, why do you need medics?" So I told him about the knife, the guns, the good possibility he would be shot, and about the jokes. "Any good jokes?" the dispatcher asked.

"I don't know. I'll take a closer listen and let you know." So I hung up the phone and moved in within earshot. As I did this, the emergency service police were pulling the EDP bar off the truck. The EDP bar basically looks like a large shuffleboard stick and is used to pin them against a wall so they can be detained. So I kind of figured this would come to a peaceful ending.

"So I got another one for you," the patient said as he gave himself another laceration on his stomach. "So this guy's walking down the street and he looks over and see this guy who looks like Adolf Hitler. 'Holy shit,' he says, 'anyone ever tell you you look just like Hitler?' Guy looks back at him and says, 'That's because I *am* Hitler. Yeah, I was frozen for fifty years after the war and now I'm back to take over the world again. Only this time, I'm gonna kill twelve million Jews . . . and three clowns.'" The patient gave a cop a nod that signified he had come to the punchline of the joke.

"I don't get it," said a bewildered cop. "Three clowns?"

"See, nobody gives a fuck about the Jews." With that, all of the officers started laughing. *The joke really wasn't funny, but the delivery!* Pleased with himself for making the cops laugh, the patient put the knife down for a moment to enjoy a laugh himself. At that moment, the ESU officers rushed him and pinned him against the wall. The other officers dove onto the pile and subdued him.

Of course, there had to be that one person who must have been watching another call than the one that was in front of her for the past fifteen minutes. Anyone who has worked in a city has encountered this person. That's the one who screams right on cue, no matter how violent the patient is, "Why you have to do that to him? Why you have to tackle him like that? He wasn't doing nuttin' to nobody." *Excuse me, who the fuck were you looking at? Do you want to take him home? I didn't think so.* It's the same no matter where you go.

My old partner JJ gave me some real food for thought one day: We are called to these people complaining that the aliens told them the government is poisoning our water supply, or the Communists at a certain hospital had brainwashed him, or even those that think they can turn themselves invisible. We laugh at them because these things seem off the wall. But wouldn't it be a kick in the ass if, when we died, we find out that it's the truth?

CELLITIS

We are dispatched to one of the police stations for a prisoner with chest pains. I walk into the holding cell area and see a nominee for next year's Best Actor Award. A middle-aged man is slumped to his right on the bench, with his hands cuffed behind his back. He is sobbing, tears and snot running down his face.

There is another prisoner sitting on the other side of the bench. He is also handcuffed. He is in much better control of himself and giving his cellmate dirty looks.

"What's the matter, sir?" I ask. *Like I really need to ask. He committed a crime, got caught, now he thinks he can get out of it by crying that's he's sick.*

"I . . . I . . . my chest hurts." He manages to say that before he starts crying again.

"What happened?"

"I . . . I was . . . my chest hurts."

A loud voice from the office behind me makes me jump. "God damn it! Be a man!" A tall, extremely built police officer with an imposing shaved head comes charging into the cell. He grabs the prisoner and pulls him to his feet.

"This is what you get for running twelve blocks from us while we were trying to arrest you. You did a man's crime, now for God's sakes, act like it! I swear to God if I hear one more whine out of you, I'll cave your fucking skull in and give you a reason to cry! Understand?"

"Um, officer?" I say calmly as I tap him on the shoulder.

"What?" He doesn't even look at me when he speaks.

"Um, I don't know how to tell you this, but you are talking to the wrong prisoner."

His eyes get very wide. He looks at the now very scared prisoner he is holding, then he looks at the quivering heap in the corner of the cell. "Well," he says to the prisoner he is holding, "just remember what I said. That goes for both you." He lets go, straightens his uniform, and walks sheepishly out of the room.

ASSAULTS

Someone once said jokingly that seventy-five percent of assault victims deserve it. I don't agree with that and think that is very insensitive, but I will go out on a limb and say there are quite a few that did something really stupid which caused them to get lumped up. Believe me, it is very hard to keep a straight face when someone is crying to you and telling you they got beat up when they know they did something dumb.

Here's an example . . .

A friend was dispatched for an assault. When he arrived on scene, he found three girls standing by a police car. They were all dressed very provocatively (and before you get mad at me for that comment, just read the rest of the story). Only one of them had injuries. She had an assortment of cuts and scrapes, and her eye was starting to swell.

"I can't believe that bastard beat me up!" she was yelling at the cops. Her friends were there to back her up, egging her on. "If I find that prick, I'm going beat his ass!" She broke down and started crying on her girlfriend's shoulder. "I don't know what happened. Why did he do this?"

"So, what happened?" My friend asked.

"Well, we met these guys at a club. We started talking to them, and decided to go back to my place. We started making out, and I went down on him. When I finished, he went down on me. That's when he found out I'm a man."

Okay, we're going to step back and take all of this case in. Let's do a little examining of the facts:

First and foremost, I am not condoning the attack, but:

1. She, or he, picked up a guy at a club that wasn't a gay club. So, it's reasonable to assume that this guy they picked up might not have been gay.

2. She tricks him into thinking she's actually a 'She' and takes him back to her place.

3. She gives him oral sex, while he is assuming that it is a female doing it to him.

4. Then, she is shocked that he got angry when he found out that She was a He? What did she expect, him to laugh and say something witty like, "Oh, you're a guy! Ha ha, well that would explain your mustache and the extra bulge in your pants!"

I was dispatched for a female with a back injury one afternoon. When I arrived, there was a man sprawled out on the floor complaining of back pain, following being assaulted. *This is the female with back pain,* I thought, *how did they make that mistake?* Then I found out.

"Sir, what happened?"

"Well you see," he spoke with a very feminine voice, which led me to believe he was gay. "I was shopping with some friends down at the corner store. My friend had something on him and forgot to pay. So the damn Arabs that run the store started calling us 'faggots' and saying that in their country they put faggots in a ditch and stone them to death!" Then he started babbling away this story about how the cops didn't care and how he was hurting everywhere.

"Do you take any medicine?"

"Yes. I am a pre-op transsexual. I am taking the hormones to make my breasts bigger and my voice higher. I should have the surgery in about a year."

"So, what hurts?"

"Well, my testicles hurt." *Sir or ma'am, no matter how nicely you ask me, I will not inspect those!* "And my back hurts, right in those bones that look like tits."

"Where?"

"You know, the bones that look like titties when you flex." *Well, I don't know who he's been looking at, but I don't believe I have titties on my back. I mean, I could be wrong, but I don't think so.*

"You mean your shoulder blades?"

"No. Those bones that look like titties."

"You mean your shoulder blades?"

"No, the back titties."

"You mean your shoulder blades."

"No, you know what I mean."

"You mean your scapula?"

"Yeah, that's it."

"Sir, your shoulder blades *are* your scapulas."

"No they're not!" *I guess I'm wrong. I mean, I only went through the equivalent of six semesters of anatomy between high school, college, and EMT class. I guess your shoulder blades aren't your scapulas!*

Anyway, we packaged him up and got ready to leave. As we were about to leave, the police showed up. After talking with the patient for a few minutes, the officer called on his radio to his dispatcher and said that he was "on scene with the twenty-six-year-old Hispanic female from the assault."

"Excuse me, officer," he said, sound rather defensive, "I am a transsexual, not a female."

"Yeah . . ." the officer said, "and fuck you. I'm not saying that over the radio." *Why would he get defensive about that?*

He wants to be a female. He's taking the medicine to be a female, granted it didn't seem to be making any difference for him, but he was trying none the less. So why get upset when someone calls him a female?

We brought the patient to the hospital, and due to the flu bug that was going around, the ER was crowded and had no beds. We had placed the patient on a back board at the scene, so we had to wait with him while they got us a bed. The nurse came over and asked what the problem was, and he started into the whole routine about how his back hurt, "right where the bones in your back look like titties. No, not my shoulder blades, the back titties."

Finally, a bed arrived and we moved him over. He looked at me and asked if I could do him a favor. I said that I couldn't because I had to go, but the nurse would be over in a few minutes to help him. That wasn't good enough for him. He started yelling for me to do him a favor. I tried to ignore him, but finally he yelled out, "Can I please have an ice pack for my testicles!"

Everything came to a sudden halt in the ER with that. I looked around and everyone was looking at me. "Why is everyone looking at me? My testicles are fine!"

I was on scene for a stabbing. I was trying to get information from my patient as we were dressing his wounds and securing him to a long board. I didn't realize that the chief was right before me, looking over my shoulder.

"Sir, are you allergic to anything?"

"Yeah, he's allergic to knives, Dick!" the chief said and walked away laughing.

Luckily, for our safety, on the majority of assault calls we get called for, we arrive after the assault has taken place. But there are several of these calls that you just wish you could have been there to witness.

I was dispatched to an office complex in Jersey City for an assault. It was on the ground floor, in the restaurant I was told. When we arrived there was a lady waving us down out in the street.

We pulled over, got out, and she began to tell us the story. She had been waiting in line at this buffet when a lady just cut her way through the line ahead of her. Well, Lady 1 was not going to stand for this. She walked up to Lady 2 and gave her a piece of her mind. And as she was describing this to me, I felt cheated that I had missed this.

In the days of chivalry, you defended an insult to your honor by challenging the offender to a duel. To do this, you slapped the offender in the face with your glove. I'm sure we've all seen Bugs Bunny do that. Well, Lady 1 decided to give it a modern twist. She picked up a Styrofoam container and smacked Lady 2 in the face.

Then Lady 2 responded by throwing down her tray and going for the salad. She hit Lady 1 in the face with a handful of shredded lettuce. Lady 1 threw a handful of tomatoes at Lady 2, who then threw a handful of cottage cheese back. Soon they are chasing each other around the buffet table with plastic salad tongs. And to make matters worse, Lady 1 was now complaining that she was hurt in the fight. Witnesses said that they never actually hit each other with the salad tongs, so what was her problem? The cottage cheese wasn't low fat? *Because I can see how that would be an emergency.*

Another call I wish I had seen firsthand happened at a laundromat. I almost got to see it, but I had to position myself up the street so that the SWAT team could get in.

We were dispatched for a head injury. Not really expecting anything odd, we pulled up right in front of the laundromat. As soon as we put the truck in park, a garbage can came crashing out through the front window of the store. Seeing there was a large-scale wrestling match inside, we decided not to enter until the police could get everything under control.

We parked up the street and tried to watch what was going on. The Emergency Service Unit and K-9 divisions of the Jersey City Police showed up within minutes of us radioing for help. The ESU suited up for a riot. Guns drawn, they stood outside and covered the exit of the store. Then, they released the dogs into the store. I always get a kick out of seeing how fast those dogs break up a crowd. People were falling over each trying to get out, one person even jumped through the broken glass.

When we went inside, the place was trashed. Clothes were everywhere, shelves were broken, and washing machines were overturned. Two adult men were the only ones injured. Here's what had happened:

A lady was washing her clothes, and some guy tried to jump ahead of her in line for the dryer. She began yelling at him, and he tried to hit her. Then, seeing that his mom was being yelled at, her seven-year-old son tried to come to her defense. He started yelling at this guy to leave his mommy alone. So what did this big, strong, macho man do? He picked the seven-year-old up and threw him across the room. The lady's boyfriend, who was oblivious at first, suddenly had to make a diving catch for his son. Am I the only one who thinks it would have been cool to see this kid get thrown across the room and his dad make a diving catch for him?

Then the boyfriend grabbed a rack of shelves and threw it across the room at the guy. Then these two big men were chasing each other around, overturning washing machines and throwing laundry detergent at each other. At some point, the boyfriend threw the garbage can over the guy's head and started punching it. Then the guy managed to get it off and threw it out the window. *Boy, oh, boy! I wish I had a front-row seat for that. Is it becoming clear to everyone why I enjoy my job?*

★   ★   ★

I was dispatched at the request of the Jersey City Police to check on an elderly man who was the victim of a strong-arm robbery. The brave, fearless desperado who robbed him knocked on the door and forced his way in when the frail old man opened the door. *Yeah, I know, a very tough crime to pull off.*

The old man said that the robber and a female forced their way in, then made him empty out all of his possessions. In doing so, they underestimated that this man whose hands were constantly trembling owned a gun. It still makes me nervous that this frail, blind, hand-shaking old man had licenses to own several hand guns and a shot gun. A scuffle ensued, and the gun went off. No one was shot, but the robber took the gun, pistolwhipped the old man, and ran off with the money and firearm.

We told the gentleman it would be in his best interest to go to the hospital. He agreed and we took him to one of the hospitals furthest away from where he lived. While we were talking to the triage nurse, my partner and I started to recap the whole story for the nurse, including the description of the actor and possible injuries he might be complaining of. The police figured from some blood on the door handles that he would have cuts to his hand.

"That's weird," the nurse said, "I just treated someone like that a few minutes ago. He's still back there." I got up and checked out the man the nurse was talking about, and sure enough, he fit the description pretty well.

I got on the phone and told our dispatcher to contact the police. By the time I hung up the phone and walked outside, the police were beginning to swarm the hospital. I gave the first officers a better description, but it did not get out in time. Another officer stopped the man, frisked him, then let him go because the officer had not heard the updated description.

When the captain found out, he was livid. "Can you clowns stop playing Keystone Cops? This ain't a Circus!" he yelled over the radio. Luckily, the man had given his real name and address to the triage nurse, so they were able to get him a little later.

As it turned out, the man wasn't the man they were looking for. However, he did have a few outstanding drug and weapons related warrants. So I like to think I made a little difference that night.

I was dispatched for another assault outside of a bar. When I arrived, I found a middle-aged lady standing by a payphone. She had a male companion with her. "What's the problem?" I asked her. She just looked at me with a puzzled expression on her face. "What's the problem?" I asked again. Still no response. I tried it in both Spanish and French, trying to get some sort of response. Nothing.

Finally, her male companion spoke. "She's deaf, she can't hear you. I can interpret for you."

Great! I thought. "Okay, sir, ask her what happened."

"What?" he said. "I can't understand you. I'm deaf too!"

Okay, so now things are getting a little ridiculous. Just to be sure they were deaf, my partner stood behind them and started insulting them—no response. Finally, I broke out a pen and paper. I started writing down questions and showing the lady. She just stared at me even more puzzled than before.

"Oh, she probably can't read that," the companion said, "she can't read English, only Spanish."

Oh, you have got to be kidding me! I thought. *Does this mean we need to find someone fluent in Spanish Sign Language, or will regular sign language do?* Luckily, the companion said that he could sign the questions to her if we wrote them down.

We made some headway, then the police arrived. The story

came out that she was assaulted and robbed four hours ago, and now we were getting the call. Apparently, the owner of the bar noticed she had been attacked and called the police.

Upon hearing the lapse in time, and apparently not being informed that she was deaf, the police sergeant asked her, "So, why didn't you just call us when it happened?"

"Because, Sarge," one of the officers said, "she's deaf. Can you imagine that 911 call? Our dispatcher screaming, 'Hello? Anyone there?' and her just breathing heavy into the phone."

I was at a hospital filling out my paperwork when a police officer came in with a prisoner. The prisoner was screaming that the officer broke his shoulder and beat him. The officer calmly said to the nurse that he was injured when he ran off on them and they had to tackle him. Surprisingly, there were even witnesses to back up the officer's story. But the prisoner kept insulting the officer and screaming, "This cracker motherfucker beat me. Fuck you, honky motherfucker!" The officer tried to calmly quiet him down, but he kept on egging him. "Fuck you, honky cracker! You broke my shoulder!"

After several minutes of this, the officer reached his breaking point. "I didn't break your shoulder, but . . ." he grabbed the guy by the back of the neck and rammed his face into the desk, "I probably just broke your nose."

Needless to say, that officer no longer is with that police force, having left of his own free will after that incident. I don't agree with police brutality, but in this case . . .

EMT Fred (not his real name) was paired up with a partner that he couldn't stand. His partner would not stop complaining. After enduring six hours with his whining partner, they were dispatched to a sick person call on the top floor of a building with no elevator and no power. Fred had a flashlight and offered it to his partner. The partner declined and began complaining about the house having no power, having no elevator, and he didn't want to walk up the stairs in the dark, and "fuck this" and "fuck that."

Fred finally broke. He was walking up the pitch-black stairs, the only sound he could hear was his partner complaining. He yelled, "Watch out!" and threw the flashlight on the ground, leaving the stairs in complete darkness. Then he punched his partner in the face, knocking him back down the stairs. Before his partner knew what happened, Fred was on the radio screaming to the dispatcher that someone had just assaulted his partner.

An ambulance was dispatched for an assault in which a Parking Authority employee was hurt. I don't care what city you are in; the Parking Authority is the Evil Empire. When I was going to college in Jersey City, classmates spent more money on parking fines than they did on tuition.

The ambulance arrived to find a Parking Authority employee complaining of having been pushed to the ground. There was an irate woman yelling at the employee that she was just waiting for her husband, and she would have moved if she was told, and a whole slew of other things.

The police arrived on scene in an unmarked patrol car and began interviewing both ladies. The ambulance got a refusal signed from the employee and were just about to leave, but something made them stop and hang around.

As the police were interviewing the lady who committed the assault, they looked over and saw that the Parking Authority lady was ticketing the undercover patrol car. Even after they reminded her that was their car, she still ticketed them.

So, what would any self-respecting police officer do in a situation like that? They took the handcuffs off the lady who assaulted the Parking Authority employee and sent her on her way. "We don't condone what you did . . . but we understand."

★ ★ ★

I was dispatched for a mutual aid call into Trenton at 3 AM for an assault. We found a young man wearing the get-up of a local gang. He was laying on the side of the road, beaten pretty badly with baseball bats.

The police had roped off the area and were trying to do an investigation. "Did you guys pat him down?"

"No, why would we do that? He's the victim."

"Well, yeah, but not to sound prejudicial, but this is probably gang related, and I don't want to take him into the hospital with weapons or drugs."

"Don't worry about that; just get him out of here," was the officer's response. So I did what I was told. We placed him on a long board and called for ALS and a trauma alert at the local trauma center. We then swiftly transported him to the hospital.

Along the way, my partner Kristen began to do an assessment of the rest of his body. We already knew he had serious head injuries, but we wanted to see what else was wrong. So she started to palpate his ribs and legs. When she pressed on his legs, he began to flinch and reach for her hands. She stopped feeling his legs, figuring he had an injury there.

As I fiddled with getting oxygen on him, he started to reach into his pants. "Get your hands where I can see them!" I yelled at him, and he listened. A minute later, he did it again. I yelled at him and he listened.

Five minutes later, we were pulling up in the ER. Security and a few nurses were waiting for us when we arrived. I was about to pull the stretcher out when I noticed the man's mask was still hooked up to the onboard oxygen tank. "Kristen, climb in there and switch the mask to the portable tank." To my surprise, she refused. "Kristen, hop in and switch the oxygen." She refused again. "God damn it, get the hell in there and switch the mask!"

"He's got a gun!" she screamed at the top of her lungs. You would have thought he had actually started shooting by the reaction that got. I tackled her, nurses tackled each other, and security guards piled on top of the patient.

"When did you find out he had a gun?" I asked her.

"The first time he reached into his pants."

"That was, like, five minutes ago. Next time, warn me then!"

It just so happened that the gun wasn't real, only a plastic cap gun. Whatever, I still can't get over the fact that the officers didn't check him.

I was dispatched for a de-watering assignment for the fire company one night. A lady called saying that the sprinklers in her apartment had gone off, and now her floor was flooded.

When we arrived, we found a good amount of water on the floor, and the sprinklers were still going off. After getting the sprinklers under control and beginning clean-up, the chief and some police officers interviewed the lady.

"I was sweeping away some cobwebs," she stated. "I saw some up by the sprinkler and began sweeping at them. I guess I swung too hard, and I set the sprinkler off when I hit it." The police seemed satisfied with that, and we were about to leave when the lady's six-year-old son came into the room.

"Mommy, you know it's not nice to lie. You know that's not what happened and you told me I should never lie."

The lady looked horrified, and the police looked surprised as well. "What happened, son?" an officer asked.

"Daddy was chasing her around with a broom; and when he swung to hit her, he hit the thing on the roof and water started coming out."

Everyone had just enough time to let that settle in when the husband walked in the front door. "Is everything all right? What's going on here?"

The police just looked at him and said, "Sir, you better come with us."

I hope someone put that kid in protective custody, because when daddy gets home. . . !

PERFECT END TO A PERFECT DAY?

The day seems to be winding down. I sit in my ambulance, reading a Stephen King novel, and listening to the waves gently batter the riverbank. It's a nice evening, and I have the window down. It's certainly been an odd day. Just another two hours and I'm off for three days. My mind starts to wander away from the book and I begin to think about how to spend the next couple of days. My eyelids are getting heavy, so I decide to take a nap.

I'm woken up by the radio. I have no idea how long I have been asleep. It takes me a moment to remember where I am. "Number 5, you need to respond to Ocean and Stegman, that's Ocean and Stegman, on the outside, for a shooting. Police on scene calling for a rush!"

I'm totally awake the instant I hear "calling for a rush." This is serious, not like the other nonsense I have been responding to all day. I hit the preset button on the radio and crank up the classic rock station. Springsteen is singing "Born to Run."

I speed up as I drive down Garfield Avenue. There's no traffic on the road. I start to get a bad feeling. I don't know what I'm nervous about, but something doesn't seem right. My left eardrum pops because of the wind that is blowing in through my open window. Not wanting to be distracted anymore, I roll up the window. Maybe my partner should have done the same thing.

The first car I see on the road refuses to pull over. I crank up the siren. I see him pull over; however, I wish I had seen the flock of pigeons. The sound of the siren causes them to take flight, at least a dozen of them. Instead of flying away from me, they head right for the ambulance.

Although it happens in a matter of seconds, it feels like it plays out in super slow motion. I hear a thump as one of the winged rats slams into the side of the ambulance. Next I see two of them bounce off of the windshield. Finally, two more make it through the open window on the passenger side. One hits the ceiling above my head, and the other flies right into my closed window. The front cab of the ambulance quickly fills up with gray feathers, and blood curdling squawks. Blood and chunks of pigeon cover me.

I am so surprised that I scream like a little girl and drive off the side of the road and right over a fire hydrant. A police car responding to the shooting witnesses the accident and pulls over to see if we need help. I stumble out of the ambulance, a mess of blood, feathers, bird shit and tears of laughter. This is truly the perfect ending to my day. *Just another day on the job, I guess.*

MOTOR VEHICLE MISHAPS

Many EMTs hate to handle motor vehicle accidents (MVAs). There is too much legality involved. Many times, the people are not really hurt and are just looking to sue someone. So, in order to not become one who gets sued, we have to carry a lot of unnecessary equipment and do a lot of unnecessary paperwork. It can be a real pain in the ass.

But I don't mind doing MVAs so much. Why? First, they are on the outside of a building (hopefully) so there is not much lifting involved. Also, people in the accident can come up with some of the most outrageous stories to get out of a ticket. Not to mention that drunk drivers can be a great source of entertainment under the right circumstances. Finally, there is the potential for outright mayhem when you go to a scene.

I was called to an MVA with entrapment in Lawrence one rainy evening. When we arrived, there were three cars involved, three people lying in the street, one sitting on the curb, and one person trapped in her car. Another ambulance arrived about the same time we did, so I was told to help the person still inside the car.

The lady was seated in the passenger seat. The door was dented so that it was pushed onto her lap. The dashboard was crumpled in such a way that it trapped her legs. I climbed in the back and held stabilization on her head. It was early fall and still warm, so I had a short sleeve shirt on.

There was another person on the scene that identified himself as an EMT. The incident commander told him to come over and help me. I had heard stories that he was a real screw up, but I believe in giving everyone the benefit of the doubt. I was still new at the time and I figured *how bad could he be?*

I told him to get a collar and set up the backboard so it was ready when they cut her out of the car. He came back a few minutes later and attempted to get the collar on the lady. He was having a hard time, and I told him to wait until they cut the car and we had more room. Then he broke one of the cardinal rules of EMS: he cut a Down Feather coat.

As soon as he did that, little white feathers filled the car like someone had discharged a fire extinguisher. Feathers all over the place, on my clothes, in my hair, in my mouth. But the weird thing was what was going through my head. Instead of yelling at him for cutting the coat and making a mess, I was thinking, *Down coats are pretty nice, I bet they'd be warm in the winter. How come mom never bought me a Down coat or comforter?*

I found out later. I was talking to the rest of the people on the call back at the station about a half-hour later. I was feeling this burning sensation in my wrists. I felt like I had glass shards in my skin. I looked down and they were covered in a rash. That's when the realization hit me, and I began to feel lousy all over. I am allergic to Down Feathers. I was covered in a rash, almost from head to toe. Everywhere I had touch after coming into contact with the feathers now had a rash. I just wish I had come to that conclusion much sooner, say, before I went to bathroom.

On another call, I found a hard top Jeep Wrangler had snapped a utility pole in half. The Jeep was sitting over the stump, and the rest of the pole was leaning on the vehicle. There was one occupant still in the vehicle. I walked near the vehicle to see if the patient was alive. He was moving around, asking if he could get out.

"Sir, it might be better if you don't move," I said. "What hurts?"

"Nothing really, just my shoulder."

The incident commander ordered everyone away from the vehicle because we weren't sure what type of utility pole it was, and he was afraid that the wires might snap. I stayed close enough to the car so that I could keep in close contact with the patient. He kept asking me if he could have a cigarette. I kept saying no because he might blow us all up, and that we'd light up at the hospital.

Public service repairmen made it to the scene, judged the pole to be a telephone pole, and that it was of no real danger to us. I climbed into the car and took up stabilization. "What's your name, man?" the patient asked me. I introduced myself. "You're the man, me and you should party sometime." I could smell the alcohol on his breath.

"Looks like you done enough partying for the both of us." He got a good laugh out of that. He started to reach for a cigarette. I grabbed the pack and flung them out the window. "Them things'll kill you. We'll light up when we get to the hospital."

"You're the man!"

"Naw, I'm just the man sitting next to the man," I said.

We finally cut the door off the Jeep and moved the patient to the ambulance. "Devin," the patient said to me, "are you coming with me?"

"You want me to?"

"Yeah, I love you, brother. You da man."

So I rode over to the hospital with him. Once we got there, he asked if we would smoke. I told him that I didn't smoke, but as soon as the doctors had seen him, he could smoke. We transferred him over to the hospital bed and cleaned up.

Just as we were about to leave, the doctor popped his head out and asked, "Who's Devin?" I said I was, and he told me the patient wanted to talk to me.

I walked in and he said, "Devin, thanks. I love you man!"

"I love you, too, man. But you ain't getting my Bud Lite!"

One of my first MVAs in Jersey City happened, or didn't happen, in the middle of a busy intersection. We pulled up, looked around and saw no accident. We drove around for a little bit and saw nothing. We drove back through the intersection and saw a car sitting off to the side of the road. Just on a hunch we decided to look at that car.

We found four people inside the two-door car. Everyone of them was complaining about having head and neck pain. Each one swore they couldn't move. And none of them knew what happened. There was no damage to the car, outside or inside. I mean, not even a scratch! A lady on the street who had been selling newspapers for the last hour said she didn't remember seeing anything. All of them wanted to go to the hospital.

The fire department's rescue company pulled up, having been dispatched as a first responder to the accident.

"What's up?" the captain asked.

"We got four people in the car, swearing they were in an accident, but there's no damage. Everyone of them wants to go to the hospital. They swear they can't move. You'll probably have to cut the roof of the car."

"Forget that!" he said. He walked over to the car, opened the door and announced very loudly, "I smell diesel fuel. Anyone who doesn't want to blow up better get out now."

I have never seen anyone move as fast as these four people did. For the life of me, I still haven't figure out what went on that night. Was there even an accident? I'll probably never know.

A friend was dispatched for a four-car pile up on the Pulaski Skyway in Jersey City. When the arrived, there was an obviously drunk man stumbling around approaching them.

The police arrived and began interviewing the drivers, including the drunken man. It came out that the drunk was the cause, and no one was injured. They began to get refusals from everyone involved. After tending to the other drivers and passengers, they turned their attention to the drunk man. Although he was drunk, he still came up with some of the best answers I have ever heard.

"Sir," my friend Dave asked, "when is your birthday?"

"August fourth."

"What year?"

"Every year."

Okay, good answer. Next question. "How much have you had to drink tonight?"

He thought for a moment, then answered, "Not enough, as you can very well tell."

Another very good answer. Now time for the final, and best answer. "Well, when was your last drink?"

"Last drink? Motherfucker, I ain't dead yet!"

I read that some major city, I think it was New York City, did a sting operation. The police staged a bus accident in the middle of a busy street. This was to combat insurance fraud. The bus was filled with undercover police officers. People climbed onto the bus, sat down, and started complaining that they were injured in the accident. About fifty people were arrested.

How stupid can anyone be? Can people get any greedier?

I was dispatched for an MVA in front the police station in Lawrence. Much to my surprise, I arrived to find the police had the patient at gunpoint.

The patient, one of Lawrence's local degenerates, decided that tonight would be a good night to get drunk. Not that that was bad, but he decided that when he was drunk, he would try to enact a little revenge on the police. So he drove his car through someone's backyard, through the fence behind the police station, and slammed into two patrol cars. He narrowly missed the brand new Expedition by a matter of feet. Then he took off and slammed into the generator building, backed up, and did it a few more times.

When the police grabbed him, he started yelling that he knew officer Bobby J. "Call Bobby J! He'll set things right." This kid learned a couple of important lessons that night. One was not to drink and drive. Another was to not drink and drive into a police station. The final, and most important one, is when you begin screaming that you know a particular officer, make sure he isn't the one you are screaming at. That sort of ruins your credibility.

My partner Wendell told me he was dispatched for an MVA with entrapment on the Garden State Parkway in East Orange, New Jersey. He found a van had rolled over and was sitting in a ditch on the side of the road.

The man driving was the only person in the van, and the van was the only vehicle involved in the crash. The man didn't appear to be that badly injured. "Sir, what happened?" Wendell asked.

"I was driving down the road, and I needed a drink. So I put the auto pilot on and climbed in the back to get a beer."

"You did what?"

"I put the auto pilot on and climbed in the back to get a beer."

"You're kidding, right? There's no such thing as auto pilot."

"Sure there is. The dealer said that if I set this switch on the steering wheel, then the van practically drives itself."

"Sir, you just described the cruise control."

"Yeah, that's it, cruise control, auto pilot. They're the same thing, right?"

Shouldn't there be an intelligence test before you get your driver's license? For the folks at home, at the writing of this book, *no auto pilot has been invented for a car.* Maybe in the future, but not right now.

Gee, I hope he wasn't stupid enough to tell the police that he went into the back to get a beer.

On a Friday the thirteenth, I was called to an MVA with an overturned car on US Route 1 in Lawrenceville. When we pulled up, we saw a car sitting upright on its wheels, banged up beyond belief. The only way we could tell what kind of car it was by looking in through the driver's side window, up through the sun roof at the hood ornament that was coming through the open window.

There was a large hole in the front windshield. And the weird thing was, there was no patient. From the damage on the ground and eyewitnesses, we were able to piece together that the car was traveling very fast, hit the curb, and flipped over. It rolled over seven times before coming to rest. The driver was ejected from the car. The bloodstains showed that he was ejected during about the third roll over. The car must have rolled over him.

The police alerted all of the neighboring police departments and hospitals to look out for him. We went back to the station. Just as we were pulling in, we got dispatched to Hamilton Township (a neighboring town) for a patient who was injured in a previous MVA and now wanted to go to the hospital. Of course it was him. The police in that town figured we would want to take him to the hospital, so they requested us instead of their own ambulance.

We found him sitting on the hood of a car from Florida. He looked very dazed. He had a few cuts and some major road rash; other than that, he looked okay. He said that he had been traveling about a hundred miles per hour on the way home to get ready for his girlfriend's prom. He hit the curb, rolled over, and was ejected because he hadn't been wearing his seat belt. He got up, a little dazed, then flagged down a passing motorist. This person was from Florida and wasn't sure of where anything was in the area. The patient asked him to take him to Hamilton Hospital and said he would give him directions. Only, his concussion made him forget his way, and so he just gave the driver directions to his girlfriend's.

A few things we can learn from this:

1. Wear your seat belt.
2. Don't do a hundred miles an hour in a fifty-five mile-an-hour zone.
3. Don't get into an accident before you go to the prom. (His girlfriend kicked his ass after that.)
4. Don't pick up hitchhikers, especially when you just saw one flip his car.

I was dispatched to an MVA in Trenton. When we arrived, we found a man holding a baby in his arms. He told us that a car came flying down the street, lost control, and struck a telephone pole. The door opened up, and the baby was thrown out. No one saw what the plate number had been, and they couldn't provide a very good description of the car except for its color and style.

When the police arrived, they informed us that a car of the same color and general description was wanted in connection with a robbery. Now more than ever they wanted that license plate number. They were getting very frustrated with the bystanders for not remembering the plate number.

I did a little exploring, then came back to the sergeant. "Sarge, here, will this help?" In my hands I had the entire front bumper, with the license plate on it.

The driver only lived a few blocks from the accident, and yes, he was dumb enough to drive home. He was found, arrested, and charged with a multitude of charges including robbery, child endangerment, and leaving the scene of an accident.

My partner Jose and I were taking a patient to the hospital one afternoon. She was only complaining of not feeling well, maybe the flu, and because it was snowing out we saw no need to race to the hospital with the lights and sirens on. As we were taking an easy trip up, someone pulled out and hit us. No damage was done to the ambulance, but the guy wrapped his car around the front wheel of the truck.

I got out to see if he was okay. Everyone in the car was wearing a seatbelt, including the one-year-old girl in the front seat that *only* had a seatbelt on—no car seat. They didn't want to go to the hospital; they said they would just wait for the police.

As per our policy, I had to get refusals signed by everyone in the car. I began by asking the driver what his name was. He gave me his name, but every time I asked him to spell it for me, he spelled it a different way. Then he refused to sign the refusal until the police showed up.

After speaking with the police, he agreed to sign. Only now, he gave me another name altogether. He said, "Oh, I didn't know what you wanted my name for when you asked before." Now I'd had enough of this joker.

The police officer came over to me and asked me for my account of what happened. After I told him, I asked him what the driver's name was. The police officer said that the driver told him his name was the name he gave me the first time. I explained to the officer that he gave me a false name at first.

The officer went back and started investigating a little further.

The driver had no license, no insurance, and the false name was handwritten on the registration. The officer impounded the vehicle and made them all walk home in the snow. Did I mention that the driver had no jacket, and was only wearing a tank top?

I was dispatched to an MVA with entrapment in Jersey City one evening. I found one vehicle was pushed onto the sidewalk, up against a fence. There was heavy damage to the driver's side of the car, and two people were trapped inside. There was a second car on the other side of the street with heavy front-end damage. Two people were standing by it. There was an ambulance on scene already, tending to the entrapped people. The chief was also there, and he directed me to check on the other two.

Both patients standing by the car wreaked of alcohol. I took one patient into the ambulance and started interviewing him. "Sir, were you the passenger or the driver?"

For the sake of conversation, I'll call him Fritz. (I always liked the name.) Fritz said, "No, I was the passenger. He was driving."

I finished interviewing Fritz and moved on to interview his friend. We'll call him Fred. "Fred, you were the driver, right?"

"No, I wasn't driving."

"But Fritz said that you were."

"Well, I don't know who was driving."

"How can you not know who was driving?"

"I never seen him before."

"You'd never seen him before, but you got in his car? Where is he now?"

"I don't know . . . he ran off."

"Well, what's his name?"

"I don't know." *This is taking ignorance to a whole new level!*

Just then, the police officer opened the door and stepped in to get more information from Fred.

"So, Fred, you were the driver, right?"

"No, I don't know who was driving. He got out and ran off."

"That ain't what your friend said," the officer stated.

"Well, he don't know what's going on. Besides, I can't drive a car. I don't even have a license."

"What? You don't have a license," the officer went on sarcastically and overly dramatic. "Well then, my mistake. How can you drive without a license? No one ever does that! Hey Mikey!" he yelled to another officer. "Get this. We must have grabbed the wrong guy. He says he doesn't have a license."

"Holy shit!" Mikey said. "Let 'em go. No one in Jersey City drives without a license." Mikey was laughing the whole time he put the handcuffs on Fred.

An ambulance was dispatched for an MVA in North Brunswick, New Jersey. When the BLS arrived, they quickly requested paramedics.

The paramedics arrived as the BLS were removing the patient from the car. The patient, an elderly lady, was secured to a long board. Her face was wrapped up in gauze bandages. The bandages were soaking through with blood.

"What's the problem?" one paramedic asked.

"This!" The EMT removed the soaked bandages and revealed that patient had nearly amputated her nose. It flapped up and almost touched her forehead.

"Ma'am," the paramedic asked, "does anything hurt you right now?"

"Well, my head really hurts, and . . ." she paused thoughtfully, "(sniff) I can't (sniff) smell too good right now."

★　★　★

During a very cold and rainy storm, an ambulance was dispatched for an MVA with entrapment on a backwoods road near Princeton, New Jersey. When the crew arrived, there was a car that had run off the road and struck a tree. The nearby canal was overflowing and starting to flood the car.

One of the crew members looked in and saw that the female patient had bright blue lips. Thinking that she was having a respiratory compromise, he called for oxygen and a rapid extrication of the patient. They pulled her out of the car and put her on a long board. She wasn't lying right on the board, so they had to readjust her. As they readjusted her, her mini skirt became caught on something and slid up, revealing that she wasn't wearing any panties. The following is how it was described to me by the guy telling me the story:

"I said 'umm!' then Scott said 'umm!' then the two medics, you know, the ones we always thought were lesbians, said 'umm!'"

Everyone got a good laugh at themselves when they pulled the male passenger out of the car. He was wearing an outfit that looked like Michael Keaton in *Beetlejuice*, the one with the white and black stripes. As it turns out, the two were on their way to a rave at a club in Trenton. The girl's blue lips that got everyone so worried . . . blue lipstick.

DON'T GET MAD, GET EVEN

This job is tough enough without the patients' attitudes making things worse. This is why I think it is important for EMTs to be level-headed and not easily rattled by what people say to them. I have worked with many people who would just as soon beat the patient than let a comment roll off their backs. But I'm here to help.

For those reading this book who are not in the business, my advice to you is to let us do our jobs. Just because you think something is the end of the world does not mean that we have to panic too. Just because we are taking our time and not running around like chickens with our heads cut off, it does not mean that we are lazy or don't care. If you call for our help, just let us help you without finding every opportunity to belittle us. Thank you.

For those on the job, here is my advice for you. Like the chapter title says, don't get mad, get creative! There are ways to exact a fulfilling amount of retribution on the patient who is a complete son-of-a-bitch. First you must ask yourself, "Is the patient acting like this because of a medical reason?" We all know that diabetes and other illnesses can cause people to act irrationally. If that is the case, just grin and bear it. The same holds true, although I've probably broken this rule before, for people with psychiatric illnesses. For the most part, they can't help the way they are. Just let them be.

Then there are the frequent flyers with no need for travel, the regular belligerent drunks, and those who are just all around assholes. The lay people reading this may be wondering what we consider an SOB or a patient who really frustrates us. Here is a brief list of indicators.

1. The patient always calls for the ambulance to take him to the hospital but then gets violent or nasty with the crew when they show up.
2. The patient constantly abuses the system by calling for a ride to the hospital so he can get a meal, a shower, a bed, whatever.
3. The patient is obviously bullshitting you.
4. The patient refuses to listen to the crew when the crew tries to calm the patient down because she is panicking for no reason.

Here are some interesting ways I have heard or seen to deal with an SOB like this. I am totally against violence or torturing a patient. However, I do advocate and welcome stories of creative stress management.

In Lawrence, we had a problem with a frequent flyer. He was a below-the-knee amputee and would call for the ambulance every day. When I say every day, I mean *every day* with the same excuse. "I had a dream that I could walk again and when I woke up I tried and fell and hurt my leg." I know that amputees can experience phantom sensations (they feel like the limb is still there), so I'm not saying that everyone with this story is bullshitting you. *But come on, every day?*

Needless to say, we would get dispatched for him and take him to the same hospital with his wheelchair. He would always be placed in the wheelchair and left in the waiting room for the triage nurse. This went on for a good couple of weeks. Then we started to get wise. We received a call from the triage nurse one afternoon asking us where we had put Mr. Hot. (I swear that's what he called himself.) After we sat in the waiting room, she told us he must have left. Then a police officer in Trenton informed us that he saw Mr. Hot wheeling himself down the street to see one of Trenton's urban pharmacists (drug dealers). All this time he was using us as a taxi so he could score some drugs.

That was it. Now it was war. The next time he called, one of our members "walked" him to the ambulance. Rather than just wheeling him out in the chair, he made Mr. Hot hop out. Two of the hospitals in Trenton were too busy and not accepting patients, so we just told him that the other one was closed, too. If he wanted to go to the hospital, we would be glad to take him to the one in Princeton, about twenty minutes away. Well, you would be surprised how quickly the pain cleared up and he signed a refusal. After that, the only time we were called for him was when he legitimately overdosed.

A person who shall remain anonymous (not me) was always being dispatched for the same lady for the same reason. She would always call because she couldn't breathe. When the ambulance arrived, they would find her talking normally, moving good amounts of air through her lungs with no problems, and there would be nothing significant showing on the heart monitor. When they took her to the hospital, all of the tests showed up negative. It was probably all in her mind. But she would not stop calling. Not every day, but maybe every other day. And the worst part was that there was someone living with her who could have driven her to the hospital all these times.

One day, they were dispatched three times for her. She

called very early in the morning and was released from the hospital. She called back around noon and was released from the hospital again. Then she called back later that night and signed a refusal. On the way out the door, one of the paramedics turned to crew and said, "I don't think she'll be calling back for a while."

"Why not?"

"Because I yanked her phone out of the wall."

Now, I know everyone is thinking how cruel that was, but don't worry, she got them back. That morning, right before the paramedic was supposed to go home, they were called back for her, for the same problem, or lack thereof. When they arrived on scene, the first words out of her mouth were, "I was trying to call you before, but my phone wasn't working. Luckily I had my cell phone." *Yeah, lucky I guess.*

One of things that really pisses us off are patients who bullshit us. Everyone should be pissed at these people. They waste our time and they keep us away from helping people who are really in need. The worst offenders are motor vehicle accident "victims." The Prudential Syndrome kicks in as soon as they realize there's been an accident, and they smell money.

This is one of the few times the rules and regulations that make our job such a hassle actually come in handy. According to our Standard of Care, there are certain things we should do. If we don't do them, our care is seen as less than adequate. So, why not go above and beyond for that patient who is bullshitting you? You can't get in any trouble for acting on the side of caution.

It's on these calls that EMTs get the angriest and let their emotions cloud their judgment. "Oh, he's bullshitting me, so I'm going to walk him."

No, you don't want to do that. Place the patient on the backboard, remember how uncomfortable they are? Take the

KED out of the truck, dust it off, and use it. Sure, it takes more time, but the look of discomfort on the patient's face will be reward enough.

I worked with a guy who was scissors happy. Anytime a patient from a motor vehicle accident would complain about any type of pain, off came the clothes. Does that sound a bit much? Well, they are supposed to be trauma stripped when you take them to a trauma center. And if he was ever asked about it in court, all he needed to say was, "How was I supposed to know what other injuries the patient had?" and everything would be fine.

One very cold, snowy evening, we had an extremely BS call. There was barely a scratch on the car. We placed the patient on a backboard, and out came the shears. In a blinding flash of steel, the man was completely naked except for a hat that my partner allowed him to place over his genitals. And since we had more than two patients from the accident, we passed him off to another crew. The guy who took the report was flamboyantly gay, which really added to the man's discomfort. Maybe next time he will think twice about trying to bullshit us.

The regular drunks that we pick up can be very trying sometimes. But it is possible to have fun with their drunken state without harming the patient physically or emotionally.

I was bored one night and in a weird mood. We were dispatched to pick up Anthony, one of our regular drunks. He was sitting on the curb and growling at us. He started to sound like the WWF wrestler "The Undertaker." So we started egging him on, having him say things the wrestler would say. We were having fun, and so was he, as well as the people watching.

We had Anthony in such a good mood that we couldn't shut up the whole way to the hospital. We had him doing Robert De Niro impressions, Al Pacino, even Hulk Hogan.

The nurses at the hospital got a kick out of it when we pulled in, opened the doors, and Anthony was dancing and singing along with David Lee Roth to "Just A Gigolo." Now whenever he sees me, Anthony starts singing that for me without me even asking.

Quick, sarcastic comments are a great way to relieve a little stress, especially when they go right over the patient's head and only your partner picks up on them.

I had a very annoying patient one afternoon. She would always call for very stupid reasons. When I say stupid, I mean she would be standing across the street from a hospital and call 911 because she didn't feel well. On this occasion I asked her what was wrong. She said she had a problem with her "shingles." I told her to call a roofer.

I was flagged down by one of our drunks on the street one evening. He was complaining that his knees hurt him. "How long have they been hurting?"

"I was at the doctor's yesterday because they were hurting."

"What did he say?"

"He thinks I have the Gout."

Something in the way he said that made feel a *but* coming on. "But?"

"But my friends just think I have water on the knee." *Well then, in that case! Why should you listen to your doctor? I mean, he only went to school for eight years. No, no, trust your friends instead.*

"Well, sir," I said, "if you only have water on the knee, why don't you blow dry it with a hair dryer?"

"Gee, I never thought of that. Do you think it'll work?"

"Of course I do!" Now, mind you, I thought that it was pretty obvious from the way I was smiling that I was only joking. Much to my surprise, the man gets up and tries to leave. I should have let him go, but my conscience got the better of me and we took him to the hospital anyway.

★　★　★

EMTs have a peculiar sense of humor, which can lead to twisted ways of torturing each other. We usually do it in fun, but many times it is to enact revenge.

I had to enact revenge one night on a paramedic. I could have reported him for his attitude, but I figured that wouldn't make me happy enough.

We were dispatched for a child that was struck by a bus. When I arrived, the kid's father just threw her into my arms. Seeing the bone sticking out of her leg, I immediately switched into the *Oh, shit!* mode. I strapped her to a long board, put oxygen on her, and began my assessment. As I was checking her for more injuries, this paramedic opened the door and said with a real attitude, "Do you need us, or can we leave?" The kid's father looked really pissed at that comment.

"Yes, I need you. Now get you lazy ass in here and earn your money." He looked at me with disgust, then climbed in with a sigh.

He didn't say anything to me for the rest of the call. I thought that was it, but he decided to push the issue. When the supervisor approached me about *my* attitude, I went through the roof. So, I set about waging a silent, personal war against the lazy bum.

I listened carefully to the radio. When I was sure he was near by, I would request paramedics for even the most BS call. ("Dispatcher, my patient says he lost consciousness," when I knew he never said that.) When this paramedic would show up on scene, depending on how I felt at that moment, I would either cancel him or have him fully assess the patient. If I got another paramedic unit, I would cancel them before they got to the scene. And if I heard a real emergency get dispatched, I would cancel them. That way I would not jeopardize other people's safety because I was angry. I could tell that by halfway through the day he had had enough, but I wasn't letting up.

The *coupe de grace* came just twenty minutes before he was supposed to go home. I was dispatched on a mutual call to one of the northernmost streets of our county. He was also dispatched, as it just so happened. He was coming from one of the southernmost streets in the county. It would take him a good fifteen minutes to get there with lights and sirens, and about a half-hour to forty-five minutes to drive back without them.

We made it up there relatively quickly and found that the patient was not in any real distress and she was going to refuse anyway. I was about to cancel the paramedics when I realized who was coming. We sat there and waited for him to drive across the county and walk up five flights of stairs with all his equipment before I said, "Oh, I didn't know you guys were dispatched. I would have canceled you."

He stormed away, started to drive back, and got dispatched for another call on the way home. He was stuck there for two hours longer than he was supposed to be. He complained to the coordinator about me. *You better believe it*. Her response to him: "Don't be so lazy!"

My friend Dave found out that his partner was allergic to cats. Not that he didn't believe her, he just wanted to see what would happen. A couple of weeks went by. He had almost forgotten, almost.

They were dispatched for an elderly lady with difficulty breathing. When they arrived, his partner turned to him and said, "Dave, something doesn't smell right."

"Yeah, it's piss," he said.

"But that's not human piss."

Dave looked down and remembered what she said. He picked the little kitty up by the scruff of its neck and held it up to her. "Yeah, cat piss!"

The cat looked at her and let out an innocent "Meow!"

She looked at him, went cross-eyed, and muttered, "You

mother(achoo!)fucker! (achoo!)" He thought it was pretty funny until she went into an asthma attack. Luckily the paramedics were right outside.

Sean told me a great way for dealing with hysterical patients who are hyperventilating. The key is to use this when there is an older family member in the house nearby, preferably one that doesn't speak very good English. This is best used on young, impressionable patients. Take a small, round breath mint and place it under the patient's tongue. When the patient starts to complain that the mint is burning, the older relative will start saying that is good (*thinking of how Nitroglycerin tablets burn under the tongue*) and the patient will calm down. You just have to tell the patient it is very expensive medicine and if she tells anyone you gave it to her you'll have to charge her for it.

Another great method of patient control is used for uncooperative patients and bystanders. Patients, especially young punks, will try to act tough in front of their friends. If the friends see the kid acting tough, they'll usually egg him on and make him act tougher. However, if they see him acting weak, they'll start making fun of him. You want the friends to be making fun of the patient, that way he'll leave with you just to get away from his friends.

So how do you do it? Hide a hard rod in the middle finger of one of your leather work gloves. When the patient starts to mouth off in front of his friends, hit him across the face with the gloves. All the friends see is him getting upset that you hit him with a glove, so now they'll start making fun of him, calling him a "wimp" or a "pussy," and he'll probably do anything you say. Either that or he'll kill you. *So use your best judgment.*

EMBARRASSING MOMENTS
AND OTHER ASSORTED TALES

We can't laugh at others until we can laugh at ourselves. And believe me, EMTs have no problems laughing at themselves.

I was dispatched to the police lock-up of Lawrence Township for an unknown medical emergency. When we arrived, there was a Latino man in the cell. He was sitting on the bed, rocking back in forth and in tears.

"What's the problem?" my partner Howie asked. The man just looked at him, the telltale sign that there is a language barrier. He tried it in Spanish. *"Que pasa?"* The man responded to that by yelling and rattling off in Spanish. Howie had to rethink his strategy. "Whoa, let's try some yes or no."

Howie was admittedly severely out of practice with Spanish, so his pronunciation left much to be desired. *"Tienes usted dolor?"* Realizing the pronunciation mistake right away, I tried to warn Howie, but he just blew me off.

The man looked at him a little alarmed. So Howie asked again. The man just looked at him with the same expression.

Aggravated, Howie asked again with anger in his voice, *"Tienes usted dolor?* Do you have any pain?"

The man looked at him again, then reached into his pocket, pulled out a dollar bill, and handed it to Howie. Howie turned to me with the same look of confusion that the man gave him. "Howie, as I tried to tell you, you were asking him for a dollar."

Two police officers showed up to assist an ambulance with a dog bite call. The dogs were still on the loose, so the more seasoned veteran armed himself with the car's shotgun. He advised the newer officer to do the same, but the rookie said he was fine.

They walked down the alley, searching for the dogs in the darkness. They were about to give up when two Doberman Pinchers came out of the bushes growling. The dogs charged at them. The veteran immediately shot and killed one, but the rookie wasn't so quick. The second dog jumped on him and pinned him to the ground.

"Take your gun and shoot him!" the veteran yelled.

"I can't! You know I have dogs."

"Fuck your dogs. Your dogs don't have rabies! Shoot him!"

But, instead of using his gun, the rookie emptied his can of mace on the dog. The dog just sneezed and got angrier. Then, defying all explanation, instead of just being humane and shooting the dog, he reached for the first thing he could find. He grabbed it, then proceeded to beat the dog to death with . . . a cinder block.

After finding this out, the other officers snuck into his squad car and replaced the shotgun with a cinder block.

Two separate drunks were brought into an emergency room in Trenton, New Jersey, one night. One was a male, and the other was a female. Because there wasn't much room, they were both placed in the same cubicle area of the hospital. The ER staff didn't think this would cause a problem since both were highly combative and needed to be restrained.

All night long, the two were yelling and screaming at each other and every one else in the emergency room. The staff was going crazy listening to these two yelling, moaning, and complaining. Late into the evening, the noises stopped coming from the room.

One of the ER technicians went in to check on the two. Much to his surprise, he found the lady on top of the guy having sex. The girl turned to him and said, "Do you mind?" Then she went back to having sex.

So much for restraints.

I was working a double one day, twenty-four hours of fun in the city streets. Everything started off fine for the second half of the shift. We got breakfast, drove around for an hour or two, napped, and didn't have any calls for the first three hours. I started to drift off to sleep when we got our first call. It was for a sick person in the Exxon Station on 14th Street. 14th Street is the exit to the Holland Tunnel.

In my daze, I mumbled that there wasn't an Exxon on 14th, but they probably meant the one on 12th (the entrance to the Tunnel). We pulled up to that gas station and the attendant informed us that there was, indeed, an Exxon on 14th. Well, to make a long story short, I was still in half-asleep when I heard my partner say something about taking the fire lane on 14th.

"Okay, whatever," was my response.

I came to just in time to see traffic approaching us at high speeds. We were driving the *wrong* way down the exit street for the Holland Tunnel. The only thing I could do was scream like a little girl and put the clipboard in front of my face. *If I can't see them, they can't hurt me, right?* We managed to pull the truck in the gas station safely and find our patient. I just grabbed the keys and drove to the hospital.

My partner was talking with the nurse and I was putting the truck back together. I turned around and saw two white shirts were walking up towards me, and they looked angry. "Where's your partner?"

"He's inside, with the nurse."

"Good," one said as he stepped forward, "he'll need her when I'm done with you guys." He looked at me with these beady eyes that seem to pierce right through you when he talks. "Who was driving?"

"Wuh —well I was, on the way—"

He interrupted me. "Shut up! You drove on the way to hospital. He drove on the way to the call. Now ask me how I know." And before I could get a word in, he said, "I got a better question, dick. Did either of you two clowns know that the Port Authority Police video tapes 12th and 14th Streets? Yeah, that's right, dick. Makes for great viewing when I can see one of my ambulances driving the wrong way up a major one-way street." He stood there glaring at me; I couldn't even look him in the face. "Go on, kid, explain this."

"He said there was a fire lane, and I had no idea he would go the wrong way up the street."

"Well guess what, genius, there ain't a fire lane! Now get out of here while I talk to your partner. On second thought, stick around. He's gonna need some first aid when I get through with him."

I followed the chiefs inside and stood in the hallway with the chief who hadn't yelled at me. I have never heard the F-word being thrown around as much as I did when he yelled at my partner.

Later on that day, we were called across the city, despite much closer units, to Provost Street for an assault. That is a major station for the Port Authority Police Department in

Jersey City, and it's right off of the entrance street to the Holland Tunnel. *Dispatchers can be so cruel.*

My partner walked over to treat the patient, and I was pulled aside by the lieutenant. He looked at me for a moment, then smiled. He took the clipboard out of my hands and put it in front of my face. "I didn't recognize you at first. Now I do!"

A friend was dispatched to do a welfare check. These calls usually come when a concerned family member can't get in touch with his or her elderly relative. Often times, these will result in one of two conditions. First, the person has left for the day without telling anyone where they went. The second is that the person is dead. This time, the person had just stepped out for the day.

On this particular occasion, the fire department was dispatched along with the ambulance. No one answered the door or the phone, so the decision was made to break in. They were able to open a second floor window only far enough to fit a small person in. Being the smallest person on scene, my friend was chosen for the task.

She climbed the ladder to the window and made the mistake of climbing in head first. The firefighters held her legs and gave her a push into the window. Another mistake she made was not looking at where she was heading. They pushed her head first into the toilet. Lucky for her, it had not been used recently. However, because her head was in the bowl, the firefighters couldn't hear her yelling for them to stop pushing.

Forcing your way into someone's house is fun, but I never seem to have good luck with it.

Medical alert calls are always fun. The only thing medical alerts seem to be good for is increasing your call volume because they always seem to go off accidentally. I have responded to only one legitimate alarm. On that call, the cat had triggered the alarm, most likely trying to get away from the smell of the body that had been laying there for two weeks. Needless to say, the alarm didn't help her.

Once I was dispatched for a medical alert that was going off. When we arrived in response, there was a car in the driveway and lights on in the house, yet no one was answering the door. The neighbors came out and were frantic, saying that Mrs. Jones must be in there because they talked with her an hour ago and she wasn't planning on going anywhere.

Now the adrenaline kicks in. I went to the ambulance, grabbed an ax, and got set to break in. The police officer, not wanting to indulge in my destructive tendencies, convinced me to wait until the dispatcher tried one more time to call. They called her, we pounded on every door, and no answer. That was it for me. I choked up on the ax like a batter about to hit a home run, took a few practice swings, got set, raised the ax above my head, and . . . dropped the ax in surprise as this little old lady opened the door as I was about to swing. She seemed upset that we kept ringing the doorbell. She just waxed the floors downstairs and she didn't want to walk on them to open the front door.

Another time, I was on a mutual aid call into Trenton for an unconscious person. When we knocked on the door, it gave and opened slightly. I could see kids running around inside. I tried to open it further, but it was jammed on something. The kids were screaming that their mommy was inside and she needed help. So I tried the door again. Still, it was stuck on something, and it wouldn't budge. I began kicking it, and ramming myself against it, trying to open it up. It wouldn't give. Finally, the patient's father came down stairs yelling at me, "She's right behind the door! Stop pushing!"

Well, she got her revenge on us in a way. I guess paybacks are a bitch, but I wouldn't know because she took it out on my partner and not me. She was combative, and not just because I slammed her in the head multiple times. She was high on something. We calmed her down, but as we were getting ready to move her, she reached up and punched my partner Scott square in the testicles.

Once inside the ambulance, we began asking her questions. "What's your name?"

"Rosemary."

"Rosemary what?"

"Rosemary Dicksucker."

"Okay, Rosemary Dicksucker. Is that hyphenated? Or do you spell that the common way?"

I may be the King of Dumb-Ass Things. I am constantly doing stupid stuff. I was dispatched to a condominium complex in Lawrence for a party with difficulty breathing. It was on the first floor, and we were having a tough time getting the stretcher into the apartment. The helpful son told me that I could probably get the stretcher in through the sliding glass door with more ease.

I figured it was worth a shot, so I pulled the stretcher around the back. He was right, it was a lot easier to slide in through the back. I had just gotten through the door when I realized that I'd forgotten something in the ambulance. I turned around to walk back through the door, and WHAM! I walked right into it.

How was I supposed to know that the son would close the door the second I walked through it? I whacked my nose pretty hard, too. I thought it was broken. I turned around and saw the son looking at me with a mortified expression on his face.

"I'm okay, sir," I said. *Like he cared.* "I'm just glad I didn't break the door."

The look on his face told a different story. He was white as a ghost, and his mouth was moving but he wasn't saying anything. I looked back at the door and saw that my steel-toed boot had broken the glass. My pants were torn, and I was starting to bleed from cuts in my knee and hand. Sheepishly, I walked out through the front door.

As I walked to the truck, the paramedics were walking up the driveway. "Oh, my god!" one of them yelled. "What the hell is going on in there? We were told it was just a respiratory emergency."

I looked down at myself and saw that I was covered in blood. "Nothing, I just did something really stupid."

As if the physical scars weren't enough, the members of my squad can be so cruel. At the awards banquet later on that year, they presented me with a roll of brightly colored smiley face stickers to put on sliding glass doors so that I wouldn't have that problem anymore.

On my first call in Jersey City, I made the classic rookie mistake. We were dispatched to one of the housing projects for a party with abdominal pain. The building was deep inside this complex, so we had to park the truck on the street and walk a short distance to the apartment. I grabbed the stair chair, and my partner followed with the jump bag and clipboard.

We walked upstairs to the top floor and found a young man lying on the floor complaining of severe pain in his stomach. He said that he had been shot a while ago, and he now had a cholostomy bag to catch the waste products from his stomach. The bag had somehow been yanked out. He definitely needed to go to the hospital, and the smell of the contents of his stomach was so overpowering, we decided to move fast. We tried to sit him in the chair, but he couldn't sit up. My partner told me to run out to the truck and get the Reeves.

I did so, running down three flights of stairs and about a hundred yards (or so it felt) to the ambulance. Out of breath (because I am out of shape), I looked quickly into the rear compartment and grabbed the bright orange Reeves. I ran back with the plastic bag in my hands, across the hundred yards, up the three flights of stairs, and burst into the room. I doubled over to catch my breath and my partner looked at me and said, "Ah, Dev. Um, you wanna bring the splint bag back to the truck and bring the Reeves, please?"

I caught my breath and looked at him, then at the equipment I'd just brought in. He was right: it was the bright orange splint bag, not the bright orange Reeves. *Whose bright idea was it to store two items that look exactly alike in the same compartment anyway?* "What do you mean he brought the wrong piece of equipment?" I looked over and saw the mother was pissed.

"I'll get it, sorry. They look exactly alike."

"You best get it now, or I'll beat you senseless." She was chasing after me with her fists waving. I thought she was serious and hightailed it out of the apartment. As I ran past her window, I could hear her and my partner laughing. That caught me off guard, and I tripped and fell flat on my face in front of a very large crowd of people.

You can say what you want about me, but at least there's never a dull moment when I'm working.

One of the most memorable "rescues" I performed didn't happen in a fire or in a horrible car accident. It happened on a trampoline. We were dispatched to a gymnasium where little children were learning how to do gymnastics.

A young girl had decided to go off by herself and do her own thing. She was jumping on a trampoline unsupervised and landed wrong, dislocating her knee.

We found her sprawled out in the center of this very large trampoline. The only way we could get to her was to crawl out to her. The trampoline was about twenty feet wide, and there was no way to get under it to keep it from bouncing up and down.

I was the smallest person on my crew, at six feet and 185 pounds. The other two guys on the crew were over six-five and 250 pounds. So this was going to be a challenge to get her off the trampoline without hurting her even more.

We began by crawling out to the center, gently sliding ourselves along. Randy and I were the first to get to her; Scott was getting the equipment from the ambulance. I took one look at her leg and couldn't help myself from blurting out, "Hey, Randy, did you see this? It must hurt!" Her knee cap was pushed up to her thigh. That outburst caught Randy by surprise and he started to laugh, causing the trampoline to bounce and the patient to start screaming again.

We finally managed to calm her down, then Scott came along. Without thinking, he walked right out into the middle of the trampoline, causing it to bounce wildly and the patient to start screaming all over again. It's hard to find good rescue help.

Sometimes I wonder if patients are worth rescuing . . . from themselves.

I was called for an unconscious person on the porch of a house in Jersey City. When we arrived, we were greeted by a group of teenage Vietnamese girls and two police officers. The girls said that they walked outside and found this man lying on their porch. I was ten feet away from him and I could still smell the booze.

I walked over to him and gave him a shake. He rolled over and started grumbling. My partner and I grabbed him under the arms and lifted him up. He started yelling that he was a Vietnam Vet and that we couldn't treat him like that, and that no one cares about Veterans.

I told him that my father is also a Vietnam Vet, so I care about veterans, but that didn't change the fact that he couldn't sleep on a complete stranger's porch. He gave me a smile and started walking to the ambulance. He looked over at the girls and smiled. "Hey, looks like we got something in common. I probably greased a few of your uncles!" He started laughing, and the girls looked pretty upset. That is, of course, until he laughed so hard his pants fell down and he tripped over them, landing in a pile of mud.

Not to make EMTs sound lazy, but we like to nap when there is down time. That's not to say all we do is sleep, but it helps to charge our batteries so we can deal with our day if we nod off when there are no calls. Also, since the pay for EMTs sucks, many have to work two jobs to get by. So when there is a little down time, and you've been working for the past twenty-four hours, it's only natural to catch a little shut eye. Naturally, administrators frown upon this activity because of how it looks. So it becomes a game: *How can we nap without getting caught?* On the whole, we generally do a good job of napping and never missing a call or getting caught. There are, however, those times . . .

Once, a co-worker was hiding in what we call the "Bedroom," a fenced off wooded area near railroad tracks that is a popular napping spot for cops and ambulances. One night, this guy decided that where he was parked was too visible, so he crossed over the tracks to get out of sight. He must have been under the impression that the rail lines were no longer in use. Much to his surprise, a slow moving, very long freight train was blocking his means of exit when he was called for an assignment. Oops.

My partner and I were napping one evening behind an abandoned warehouse. It was a secluded spot, tucked away from civilization, and it was raining so we weren't that worried about someone messing with us while we were asleep. The ambulance I was in is one of the most uncomfortable places to try to sleep. There is no leg room for a guy who is six feet tall to sit comfortably, let alone recline. So I propped my legs up on the dashboard.

We napped for about a half-hour until we were called for a possible stabbing that was a mile from where we were. My partner didn't know where the street was exactly, so I hopped out of the passenger seat and went to drive. As soon as I opened the door and stepped out, I came to the realization that my legs were asleep. I fell right into a puddle of mud and flopped around like a fish trying to get myself up.

When we arrived on the scene, there was no patient. But the chief was there, and he had a few questions and comments about the mud that was caked onto my uniform.

My friend Dave told me that one day he had this overwhelming urge to overstock his truck. He placed about six long boards on the truck, when we usually only carry about four. "Ready for that bus full of nuns to crash?" is usually the question asked when someone stocks a lot of collars or long boards on the truck. He couldn't explain it; it was just something he felt he should do.

Well, luckily for the Catholic Church, no busload of nuns flipped over that day. However, the next day, those long boards would come in really handy during a heavy rain storm. Dave had the next day off, but the crew thanked him for stocking up.

It was summer, and we had one of those freak summer storms that pop out of nowhere, flood the place, then disappear within a half hour or so. This one lasted about an hour, but since it was a very slow morning, the poor ambulance crew in Dave's truck didn't realize it had rained until it was too late.

They had been napping in another secluded area that was off in a field, out of sight. They received a call for a serious emergency, stepped on the gas, and found themselves stuck in the mud. They tried to back it up, drive it forwards, everything, but they couldn't get out. So they opened up the cabinet for the long boards, and *jackpot!* They placed long boards under the wheels for traction. They finally got out, but not before they lost a couple of the long boards. I would have paid good money to see those boards shoot off into the woods like rockets. I'm sure they're still back there. Maybe one day I'll go look for them.

My friend Jen was placed in a very embarrassing situation one night. She was responding for a patient in cardiac arrest. She arrived as the paramedics were treating the patient. They looked up, tossed her the keys for their truck, and said "Drive."

So her partner drove the ambulance like he does on every call, the paramedics worked on the patient, and Jen was left to drive the paramedic truck. Now, keep in mind three things: Jen had never driven an ambulance before, had no idea how to work the radio or who to call for help, and she was new to the area. *A great recipe for disaster!*

Her partner, forgetting that she had no idea where anything was in the area, took off without seeing if she was following. She lost sight of him, then she became completely lost in downtown Trenton.

After driving around aimlessly for fifteen or twenty minutes, and on the verge of a nervous breakdown, someone finally called over the radio, "Will the EMT from Lawrence that is driving the paramedic truck please meet the crew at Helene Fuld Hospital. Or, if you are lost, just return to your building and meet them there."

So for the paramedics out there who are so quick to give your keys to the EMTs and have them drive your truck, do some careful screening before you turn it over. It's not wise to get them lost in the middle of the 'hood with a fortune of narcotics in the back of the truck.

★   ★   ★

You would think EMTs and paramedics would know better. My brother is deathly allergic to bee stings, yet he doesn't carry an Epi-kit.

One day a bee stung him while he was pulling the stretcher out of the ambulance with a patient on it. Luckily, he was at the ER.

He didn't have the normal immediate reaction of wheezing and burning, so he thought that maybe he wasn't really stung. He had calmed down and was about to leave the hospital when a nurse approached him. "Sir, are you feeling okay? You're really sweating."

At that, Sean collapsed onto the floor in a wheezing fit. Sure, I feel bad about laughing at him for that, but he should know better than to not carry his kit.

There is something about being dispatched for a child in real distress that really gets your adrenaline going. Maybe it is the feeling that a child should be given every opportunity to live, or maybe it is just the basic survival instinct in all of us to protect the young. Whatever it is, it gets us and the ambulance moving faster.

Wendell was dispatched for a "baby with trouble breathing" one night. He raced over to the house, the fire department first responders racing right behind him. When they arrived on scene, they were pounding on the doors trying to get in. Just as they were about to break open the door, a ninety-five-year-old lady opened the door, holding herself up with her walker.

"Where's the baby?" they asked her frantically.

"My baby's in his room." She pointed them to the bedroom.

They raced up the stairs and into the room. Much to their surprise, "baby with trouble breathing" meant a seventy-five-year-old man with a cold. The old lady didn't give the dispatchers time to properly screen the call. She just said her baby was having trouble breathing and hung up.

★　★　★

My partner Wendell is so afraid of dogs, it's funny. We responded to a housing project for a sick person call. We knocked on the steel door. No one answered, but a dog started barking from the other side. Wendell screamed and ran out of the building, leaving me standing alone like an idiot in the hallway.

On another occasion, we responded to a person's house. He only needed to see the carrying case for a small dog and he was running down the stairs before I could turn around and say anything to him. When I looked around, he was at the bottom of the steps cowering. I treated the patient with the help of the paramedics and we brought her out to the ambulance. I told him I would write the report if he drove to the hospital. No problem, he said, and started to get out of the back. He jumped back in and slammed the door.

"It's huge! It's this big!" He held his hands apart to gesture a large dog. "Fangs this long, and claws this big with the look of blood lust in its eyes, and the stench of death on its breath." I looked out the window and there was a guy walking his Chihuahua.

Wendell responded to a call for a man with chest pains. The paramedics were already on scene treating the patient. They had stuck the man with IVs, given him medicine, and were doing other things. All the while, his very old hound dog was asleep at the top of the stairs. He merely picked up his head when the medics walked in. But of course, when Wendell, the one person deathly afraid of dogs, comes to the house, the dog jumped up and walked over to him. Wendell threw down the equipment and ran back into the ambulance.

An ambulance was pulling into a gas station to fill up. They were approached by the attendant who said there was a man having a seizure around the corner. The ambulance went over to help him.

The man was just coming to when the attendant informed the crew that the man had just robbed him at gunpoint. After getting the money, the man had a seizure. Why did he have a seizure? Well, one reason was because he didn't take his medicine that day.

Now, I ask you, if you are going to commit any type of crime, and you know you have seizures, why not take your medicine beforehand? Do you *want* to get caught?

SIGNS YOU KNOW YOU'RE A WHACKER

Whackers are the groups of people that are at the brunt of everyone's jokes in the emergency services. These are the people that when you look at them you say, "Gee, you have no life!" Truth be told, there are those who are dedicated to the service and there are Whackers.

But how do you recognize one? Here is the signs you know you're a Whacker. While only people in the service may find these funny, if you are not in the service and recognize these signs in a loved one who is: get them help! Immediately!

· You have every radio frequency in your county memorized.
· You have memorized every dispatch tone in your county.
· Your eyes glaze over and you begin to salivate when your squad's dispatch tone goes off.
· You know the make and model of every piece of apparatus in your county.
· You know the year-end statistics for every one of your local departments.

- You own a police/fire scanner for your bedroom, one in your car, and one that is handheld.
- You carry your department pager on you even when you are too far out of range to pick anything up.
- You have the entire five-page list of radio codes for the Fire Department of New York memorized, you are not an employee, and yet you try to work them into ordinary conversation.
- You own a personal pager that tells you where every fire or major accident is around the country, and you announce to everyone around when there is a major event three states away.
- You have left in the middle of a date or having sex to answer a call.
- You have more than one blue light on your personal car.
- You have only one blue light on your car but it is bigger than the lightbar on most police patrol cars.
- You have responded to someone's call in your personal car, just to watch.
- You have so many department stickers on your back window that you can't see out.
- You have only one sticker on your back window but it is either a bulldog with a firefighter helmet, the Tasmanian Devil with a fire ax, or Calvin pissing on a fire.
- Your entire wardrobe is made up of EMS/Fire T-shirts.
- You can't wait until you get your next issue of the Gall's catalog.
- You leaf through the pages of the EMS product catalogs before you leaf through the Victoria's Secrets catalog.
- You refer to volunteering as "going to work."
- You sit around and wish for "The Big One."
- You talk like every call you went on was "The Big One."
- You own a car that looks like an undercover police car and outfit it with a spotlight on the driver's side door.
- You belong to multiple volunteer departments and wear

pagers for every one on your pants at the same time.

· You have more equipment on your belt than Batman.

· You've ever entertained the thought of gaining more weight so that you could carry more equipment on your belt.

· You have more equipment in the trunk of your car than most fire trucks do.

· You spend so much time at the station that your family forwards your mail there. The department has given you your own garage door opener and has started demanding rent.

· You bought your own set of turn-out gear and carry it in your car, just in case.

· You own a complete video collection of *Emergency* and *Rescue 911* and memorized every line in *Backdraft*.

· You take classes for topics you'll never need, like ice water rescue when you live in the desert.

· You answer everyone with "affirmative," "negative," or "stand by," even in regular conversation.

· You wear your uniform even when you are not on duty.

· You wear your department-issued leather, steel-toed boots when you go out in public because you never know when a call will come.

· You sleep at the station more nights during the week than you do in your own house.

· You arrange your clothes at the foot of your bed just in case a call comes in the middle of the night.

· Your fine dining wear is complimented by your collection of mugs and beer steins from all the parades and housing ceremonies you have attended.

· You've gone to the Firefighter's Convention in Wildwood, New Jersey, for the expositions, *not* the four-day party.

· You see making the department's Top Ten Responder List as more competitive than trying out for the Olympics.

· You've turned down invitations to go out because you had

a feeling there would be calls that night.

· You view volunteering for a duty night as your major source of social interaction for the week.

· You still wear a "Coed Naked EMS [or Firefighting]" shirt.

· You saved money on your wedding by being driven around in the back of a ambulance instead of a limo.

· You have any of the following bumper stickers on your personal vehicle:

"My other car is an ambulance"

"Honk if you know first aid!"

"I save lives, what do you do?"

"Volunteers do it 24/7"

"I'm a volunteer EMT, who the hell are you?"

· You yell into the radio every time you use it.

· You talk more on the radio than you do in regular conversation.

· You sit around writing a book about EMS.

How do I know so much about Whackers? Well, that's because I am a recovering Whacker. I'm not proud of what I used to be, but I'm not ashamed to admit it. I used to have a riding-three-nights-a-week-and-answering-four-hundred-calls-a-year habit for my volunteer squad. *Excuse me for a moment while I wipe the tears away from my eyes and compose myself. . . . Okay, that's better.* Admitting you have a problem is always the first step to recovery. So, please, if you see this behavior in someone you love, intervene. I'll be forming a twelve-step program called Whackers Anonymous in hopes of breaking this terrible, debilitating habit.

ON THE MATTER OF STRESS

Now that you've read my outrageous stories and are probably thinking it's all fun and games out there, I'm here to say it's not. (Well, not entirely!) In all seriousness, I have fun doing my job; I wouldn't have stuck with it as long as I have if I didn't enjoy it so much. But there are times when the job sucks.

If anyone tells you he or she is not bothered by at least one thing they encounter on the job, you can call them a dirty liar. And tell them I said so. (But do me a favor and wait until *after* they buy my book—thanks!) Unless you are completely devoid of all human emotions, it is impossible to do this job and come away unscathed.

I jokingly say that trying not to laugh in someone's face is the greatest on-the-job stress. It is difficult, believe me when I tell you it's difficult, but it's certainly not the hardest part of EMS.

What are some of the job stressors, you ask? (If you didn't, just humor me.)

The Nature of the Beast:

The purpose of emergency medical services is to deliver emergency care to the sick, injured, dying, or already dead. It is hard not feel something for the patients or their families. It is also difficult to not contemplate your own mortality. I think it is just human nature to feel empathy for someone in need.

Empathy can be a good thing, enabling you to treat the patient with respect. When we lose that part of ourselves, we start acting like robots. Many of my patients have commented to me about how caring other EMTs have been to them. It seems that a little bit of respect, caring, and professionalism can go a long way.

Caring becomes a problem when empathy turns into sympathy. When the EMT becomes sympathetic, it breaks down that wall of detachment we need to maintain. All too often, EMTs allow the problems of their patients to become their own. Emotional attachment and commitment should end when the patient is transferred to the care of the hospital or he signs a refusal form.

Physical Exertion:

A major part of the job is getting to the patient and moving the patient to the ambulance. Many times we must walk up insane amounts of stairs with heavy equipment, then walk back down those stairs carrying the equipment *and* the patient. In a perfect world, everyone who was sick would be the same size, shape, and waiting for me on the ground floor. But this isn't a perfect world, or else I would have legions of adoring fans singing my praises wherever I go. (Hey, a guy can dream, can't he?)

Physical Harm:

Anytime you doing any sort of lifting, you run the risk of injuring yourself. However, that's not the only way we can get injured on the job.

Diseases:

Whatever nasty bug the patient has, we're exposed to it. Unfortunately, some of the most contagious or dangerous diseases are the most embarrassing for the patient to admit. Scabies, lice, Herpes, and AIDS are some of the more commonly left out ailments. These usually come to our attention after we are exposed to it.

Unsafe Structures:

Have you ever stepped on a staircase and felt how soft or spongy it was? Eventually it has to give way, usually under a concentration of weight, like maybe two rescuers carrying thirty pounds of equipment and a 250-pound patient.

Whatever caused the person's injuries could still injure the rescuer. These include electrical currents, slippery floors, hazardous materials, and—my favorite—ice rinks.

Violence:

We're the good guys, right? The knights in pressed uniforms riding in on flashing ambulances to save the day, aren't we? Well, that all depends on who you ask. If someone is pissed off enough to beat his girlfriend, chances are he's pissed enough to beat you. There is no predictable behavior pattern for emotionally disturbed persons. Therefore, even the regular who is always calm when you pick her up has the potential to get violent. Distraught family members can attack you for not working up to their expectations. Finally, drug addicts, particularly heroin users, tend to become very nasty when you kill their high. Even if you just brought them back from the dead, they will be fighting mad that you took away their $20 high.

The Quick Pace:

I get off on the fast paced nature of the job. I can't stand doing nothing at work all day. Don't get me wrong, easy money is the best kind. But since I have the attention span of a gnat, I get cabin fever very easily and eventually run out of things to do. The down side to being busy is that the ambulance becomes your office for the day.

If you've never been in an ambulance before, let me tell you, it's cramped! Maybe not for someone who is shorter than five feet, four inches. However, it gets a lot worse as you get taller. I'm a six-footer and I drive around all day with my knees in my stomach. What's worse is that I constantly whack my head on the ceiling in the back of the truck.

It's a catch-22. I complain that I'm cramped, but as soon as I get out to stretch, I get bored and wish for calls. I know I drive my partners crazy, but it's not my fault I have no attention span. Blame television!

Another problem with always being on the go is trying to find the time to eat or take potty breaks. In the system where I work, we have to tell the dispatcher over the radio when we want to take a 'personal.' So basically, I am announcing to everyone that I have to take a crap. That bothers me. I don't want to know when everyone else is going to the bathroom, and I'm sure they don't care when I go to the bathroom. What's worse is that now I have this fear that if I take a little too long, everyone will just assume that I have a case of the runs.

Language Barriers:

It's frustrating trying to deal with patients who don't speak English. I don't believe that it is necessary to be completely fluent in English to live in America. After all, think back to how bad you or your friends did in Spanish class in high school. It's difficult to have to learn a second language. But since it is the official language, you should know enough to get by. Especially when your life depends on it!

I bought a pocket English to Spanish medical dictionary. I thought this would be the answer to all my communication woes. It had questions for every conceivable medical situation. I now know how to ask someone if his erection is stiff enough. (Which, incidentally, I am using to gauge my time here on earth. The day I have to ask a patient that is the day I hurl myself in front of a train.) On one side of the page is the question in English and the phonetic pronunciation in Spanish. On the side is the question in Spanish in large type so the patient can read it. They are all simple yes or no questions. Sounds easy enough, right? *Wrong!* Even with the phonetic spelling, I slaughter the questions beyond comprehension, and none of my patients seem able to read the questions.

Interacting with family and bystanders:

Some people have this idea that the ambulance is there solely for them. That all we do is wait around the building for that one person to call us. That's simply not true—we're not allowed to watch TV. No, seriously, it is likely that more people call for an ambulance at the same time than there are ambulances to take those calls. So, unfortunately, some people have to wait. As a result, many people take the delayed response to mean that we are lazy or don't care when, in fact, we have been working extremely hard all day.

Some people have this completely asinine notion that we can somehow make it through the day without eating. Normal eight-hour jobs provide for an hour lunch break that no one can interfere with, as well as fifteen minute coffee breaks throughout the day. I don't get a lunch break, and those of us that do can be yanked from our break at any time. Therefore, we eat as soon as we get a chance. But there is always that one asshole who has to come up to you and say, "How come you in here eating when people are out there dying?" Well, genius, if I'm eating, that means that no one needs the ambulance right now.

Is it possible for someone on the street to come up to an ambulance and *not* say something stupid to the crew? Please, I would like for one time, just once, to have someone come up to me and tell me they appreciate the work I do without that statement being followed by "Got any change?"

Driving:

My greatest stressor. I love driving because I feel like I am in control. At the same time, I hate driving because of all the idiots on the road. Everyone thinks they are the most important thing on the road. Despite being the law in many states, and just plain old fashion common courtesy, many drivers see no reason to pull out of the way for an ambulance.

How hard is it to get out of the way in a controlled manner? Just direct the car to the right. I can understand certain small streets or gridlocked traffic, but I get pissed off at taxis who cut me off, double parked cars, and people who pull to the left instead of the right.

I firmly believe that everyone should be required to ride along with an ambulance before they get their driver's license just so that they can see how frustrating it is.

Pay:

It's almost an insult how little we get. In many places, non-skilled labor gets paid more than we do.

Management:

It's awfully hard to motivate someone to work hard when management offers little or no support. "EMTs are a dime a dozen," the bosses have been known to say. That may be true, but competent, hard working, self-motivated, and professional EMTs are hard to find.

Believe it or not, EMS is a thankless job. It's important for management to make the worker feel appreciated because Lord knows the public doesn't.

So what can be done to combat this stress? Here are some of my suggestions:

Philosophy:

There are certain givens that, once accepted, will make the work experience a little less stressful.

· This job is stressful; allow it to be. There is nothing wrong with feeling pressure.
· Everyone dies; the only question is when. While this is a pessimistic attitude, it helps to get over the feelings of 'it wasn't his time!'

Saving lives is great, but that's not my job. Anyone in EMS knows that you don't save lives every time the ambulance rolls. I feel that the main purpose of this job is support. We provide emotional support as well as medical support. Even if you don't save the patient, you can still help the patient's friends and family.

Talk:

Verbalize how you feel. When something bothers you, complain. Maybe nothing will come of it, but it may help you to feel better.

Punch Out When it's Time:

There is no shame in walking away from the job when it gets to be too much. Life is too short to waste your life in a job that brings you no satisfaction. When that happens, it may be time to look elsewhere.

Party:

Any time you put four or more EMTs in a room together, complete mayhem ensues. Have fun with the people you work with. The more time you spend together, the more laughs and inside jokes you can share at work, thus making it more pleasurable.

Every year, a group from my volunteer squad goes to see Jimmy

Buffett in concert in Camden, New Jersey. This is our chance to escape our lives for a day and completely unwind. We go all out: tons of food, loud decorations, plenty of alcohol, and a tiki bar we build in the parking lot. Maybe this isn't the escape that appeals to everyone else, but find one (or more) that's right for you.

Hobbies:

Provide a balance to your life. If you work in a dull job, have adventurous hobbies. If you work in a highly stressful environment, have calming hobbies. I took up teaching myself musical instruments when I got stressed out. So, after six years, I can play the guitar, piano, harmonica, drums, and am working on the steel drums. (Can you tell I get a little stressed out on the job?)

Vacation:

Got vacation days? Use them! Not to work on your house. And don't save them. Use them now. Not all of them, but take a vacation at least once a year.

Where to go is entirely up to you. But may I make two suggestions? One: get away from civilization. Some of the most relaxing getaways I have taken were to a friend's camp in western Pennsylvania and to my girlfriend's house in Vermont. Get away from the major elements of your job for a while. Two: Experience Island Time at least once in your life. I was sitting on the beach in Nassau, Bahamas, with a margarita in hand, Herman Wouk's *Don't Stop the Carnival* open on my lap, and the Beach Boys singing "Sloop John B" on my CD player when I discovered that magical feeling of Island Time. Far away from the pressures of work, the cries for help, the wailing of the siren, and the horrible odors, sitting on a tropical island, time stands still. Nothing else matters when all you have to worry about is what drink to try next or whether or not to reapply the sunblock.

This job could arguably be one of the most stressful jobs in the world. But it doesn't have to be. Neither does yours. Find out what works for you and go with it.

THAT'S A WRAP!

There you have it, some of the highlights of the past six years of my life. I hope that you enjoyed reading this. I know I had a blast writing it. I think it's good to sit around and talk about the fun times. Life is more pleasant when we concentrate on the good times rather than the painful moments.

For those reading this who are involved in EMS: I hope that you got the most out of this book. As I said in the introduction, storytelling is a time-honored tradition in the service. As I am sure you have learned, people in emergency service jobs have some of the most twisted senses of humor known to man. And with good reason! It's hard not to see what we see on a regular basis and remain "normal." But I hope this book makes you feel that there is at least one person (me) who is more screwed up then you.

To those reading this with family or friends involved in EMS: Does this shed any light on why your loved ones love the job so much? It's also important for family and friends to understand the rollercoaster ride that is our job. It is often difficult to go from one call in which someone is dying to another call where the person makes you laugh, and then back to a life-or-death call, and then home and lead a normal life. But most of all, I hope that this book interests you enough to go to those loved ones in EMS and ask them what stories they have. Everyone of us has them, and everyone of us is dying to tell them.

And finally, for those who have no ties to EMS, but just picked this book up because it looked good: I hope this book makes you more interested in EMS. If you ask yourself, "What's going on in there?" the next time you see an ambulance go by, then I am satisfied that I did my job. EMS is a vital part of the community, but one that I feel people don't really know a lot about. Maybe this book will get some of you interested enough to find out more.

EMS has been good to me. It helped to shape me into the person I am today, helped in getting me a scholarship to college, and provided me with great memories. But, best of all, it's enabled me to meet some of the most interesting people.

I'd like to take this opportunity to thank everyone who made this book possible, either by telling me stories, or becoming the basis for them. Forgive me if I forgot anyone or misspelled someone's name.

Wendell T. Green, Dave Martinez, James Johnson, Jose Aviles, Brian Heffernen, Henry Solares, Rosa Burgos, Harry Baker, Chris Marciniak, Donnie Komlos, Eric Rush, Tito Rodriguez, Gerry Fuentes, Gerry Greene, Joe Bohrer, Gene Ryan, Carla Sanchez, Antoinette Jensen, Anne-Marie Cleary, Rich Gorman, William Newby, Steve Viuad, Daniella Maldonado, Rich Nueroter, Steve Assadourian, Justin Marguiles, Virginia Ferrara, Miguel Guerraro, Dave Bonacarte, Mickey Slattery, Joe Slattery, Mike Carrig, Dawn Macri, Chris Fink, Mike Alessi, Jen Fragaile, Lawrence Brooks, Damaris Rivera, Steve Kantera, Nancy Rivera, Julio Rivera, Pablo Lopez, Pedro Reyes, Mario Bantilan, Edgar Pitao,

Danny Polo, Ron Blothelo, Jay Bowles, Timmy Prahm, Beth Brdnjar, Steve Job, Yasmine Yaghooti, Joe Bragg, Frank Aggrassino , Myra Stith

Mike Yeh, Dave Burns, Bob Brackett, Ray Nagy, Butch Bentley, Andrew Condrat, Don Huber, Clyde D'Angelo, Tom Everist, Tom Brophy, Kevin Reading Sr, Bryan Gibbons, Mike Burns, Robin Bowden, Rich Soltis

Scott Stein, Anne Stein, Meggin Stein, Marc Poveromo, Alexis Durlacher, Sue Fabian, Lisa Fair, Aaron Van Hise, Carol Bastian, Jason Pidcock, Randy Wagner, Howie Sislin, Chris Dimeglio, Dolly Dimeglio, Tara Conover, Joanne Tobiasz, Rick Evans, Chrissy Vincent, Maryanne Russell, Mike Peterson, Kristen Behnke, Dave Miele,

Joe Vallo, Charity Grieco, Ed Bialowlogski, Brett Levine, and Barry Erlbaum, and anyone else I may have forgotten.

To my family: Mom, Dad, Brian, and Brendan. Especially to Sean for being a role model of EMS for me, and for providing me with a ton of New York City stories.

To Erin Belz for being an incredible friend and for planting the idea that became this book.

And finally, to Jen Goralski. Without you, I might have given up on the idea before I started. Thanks for always pushing me, for constantly reading over my shoulder, and for being my pillar of support.

EMS TERMS AND ABBREVIATIONS

Emergency medical service personnel have one of the most colorful work languages. It may vary slightly from region to region, but it's just about the same all over.

ABC: According to the textbook, it means *Airway, Breathing, and Circulation.* This could be the most important assessment tool for the EMT. Basically stated: is the person breathing and do they have a pulse?

Actor: The person who commits an assault.

AIDS: *Acquired Immunodeficiency Syndrome.*

ALS: *Advanced Life Support,* paramedics. They are capable of administering medication, IVs, and other advanced life saving techniques.

AMS: *Altered Mental Status.*

The Bag: A kevlar body bag carried by some police departments, used as a restraint for violent patients.

Banged Out: (1) to be dispatched for a call; a.k.a. tapped out, paged out, hit out. (2) to call in sick.

Bird: A helicopter; a.k.a. chopper, life-flight, Medivac.

BLS: *Basic Life Support,* are usually dispatched on all types of calls; cannot administer medications, IV, etc. These units are usually the transportation unit.

BP: *Blood pressure.*

Bus: A term for an ambulance, usually because we feel like we just bus people around all day.

BVM: *Bag-Valve-Mask;* a mask with a plastic bag on the end that you squeeze; used to deliver oxygen into a person who is not breathing.

C-Spine Precautions: Measures taken to protect the cervical spine of patients who may have injured their backs. These include, but are not limited to, a cervical (neck) collar and a long board.

CAD: *Computer Aided Dispatch.*

Cadet or Junior: A volunteer member who is under the age of 18 years of age.

CAOx3: *Conscious, Alert, Oriented x 3;* the patient is awake, talking to you, and can tell you who, where, and when he is.

CHF: *Congestive Heart Failure;* a condition characterized by the patient's lungs filling up with fluid.

CO: *Corrections Officer* or *Carbon Monoxide.*

Code: A cardiac arrest call, or to go into cardiac arrest. *Proper use:* "He coded on us," or "Respond for the working code."

Code Blue: In the Emergency Room, signifies that a patient in cardiac arrest or critical condition is coming into the ER, or that a patient went into cardiac arrest.

COPD: *Chronic Obstructive Pulmonary Disease;* a disease that interferes with breathing. Emphysema.

CPR: *Cardiopulmonary Resuscitation.*

CVA: *Cerebralvascular Attack;* a stroke.

Dip: A mixture of marijuana, PCP, and formaldehyde. Yes, some genius figured out you can smoke pot laced with embalming fluid.

DNR: *Do Not Resuscitate;* a legal document expressing the patient's wishes to refuse certain procedures which would prolong his/her life in the event that they are rendered unconscious or unable to make such a decision, with no hope of recovery.

DOA: *Dead on Arrival.*

Dope: Can mean a variety of illegal drugs, including heroin, marijuana, or cocaine.

Drop A Line: To start an IV.

E-911: *Enhanced 911;* computers that better track where a 911 call is coming from.

EDP: *Emotionally Disturbed Person;* the politically correct way of saying a person is mentally ill.

EMT: *Emergency Medical Technician.* They are trained in various basic fields including, but not limited to, first aid, CPR, airway management, and splinting of injured limbs.

Epi-Pen (or kit): A small, needle-like device that injects the medicine epinephrine into a person's body to counteract an allergic reaction to a bee sting.

ER: *Emergency Room.*

ESU: *Emergency Service Unit;* a police rescue/SWAT team, used extensively by police departments in the New York area. (a.k.a. *E-Squad*)

ETA: *Estimated Time of Arrival.*

EtOH: A drunk person (from the chemical formula for alcohol).

Extricate: To remove a patient from an entangling situation, i.e. car wreck, building collapse, etc.

FD: Fire department.

GOA: *Gone on Arrival*; the patient has left the scene before you get there.

GSW: *Gun Shot Wound.*

HAZMAT: *Hazardous Materials*; a group of materials, or incident involving materials that are hazardous to your health.

Haldol: A wonderful medication for psychiatric patients. Sometimes we wish they could spray the streets with it like we were spraying for mosquitoes.

HBV: *Hepatitis B Virus.*

HCV: *Hepatitis C Virus.*

HIV: *Human Immunodeficiency Virus.*

Hump: To be very busy. A simple formula to tell if you were humped: if you average one call for every hour you work, you've been *humped.* If you have more calls than hours worked, you've been *violated.*

ICU: *Intensive Care Unit.*

IP: *Intoxicated Person*; a drunk.

Jaws of Life: Hydraulic cutting, spreading, and prying tools used to extricate victims of car accidents, building collapses, etc.

Job: A call. A "Hot Job" is an exciting call, namely a shooting or a stabbing.

Jump Bag: The bag in which you carry most your important equipment on a call

Jumper: A suicidal person threatening to jump.

L & D: Labor and Delivery; when babies are born (hopefully).

LOC: Level of Consciousness, or *Loss of Consciousness.*

MCI: Mass Casualty Incident; a call with a lot of patients.

MDT: Mobile Data Terminal; computers mounted in emergency vehicles that are linked to the dispatch center.

ME: Medical Examiner; the coroner.

MI: Myocardial Infarction; a heart attack.

Mobile Crisis: A team of psychiatrists that make house calls to EDPs in need.

MOS: Member of Service; a person who is a member of a police/fire/EMS department.

Mutual Aid: When an ambulance or fire truck from one area responds to a call in someone else's area, usually because there aren't enough ambulances or fire trucks to handle the calls.

MVA: Motor Vehicle Accident.

MVA with Entrapment: A motor vehicle accident in which the patients are trapped in the car.

Narcan: A medication administered to people using heroin to counteract the drug.

NC: Nasal Cannula; a small tube that delivers a small amount of oxygen to a patient through his/her nose.

Nitro: Nitroglycerin; administered in the form of a pill, a spray, or a paste. It expands the blood vessels to help lower blood pressure and relieve chest pain.

NRB: Nonrebreather Mask; a mask with an inflatable bag

attached to it; used to deliver a large amount of oxygen to patients who can still breath on their own.

O2: Oxygen.

OB/GYN: *Obstetrics and Gynecology.*

On the Job: An expression used to mean that someone is a police officer, firefighter, or EMT. *Proper use:* "He's on the job in New York City."

OR: *Operating Room.*

PD: *Police department.*

Per Diem: A person who works part time.

PO: *Police Officer.*

Priority of Response: 1: A life threatening emergency, use lights and sirens and hurry. 2: A non-life threatening emergency; use lights and sirens but don't kill yourself to get there. 3: Not really an emergency at all, or the emergency has been mitigated; don't use lights or sirens.

Probie: A person who is new to the department and on probationary status.

Put A Rush On: To hurry up the unit. *Proper Use:* "Police are telling us to put a rush on the bus!"

Radio: A police patrol car.

Rales: The crackling sound made in the lungs when they fill up with fluid.

Recovery: An operation to remove a dead body from a scene, i.e. a car wreck, confined space, etc.

Reeves: A type of carrying device that wraps around the patient and enables the rescuer to carry a patient down the stairs in the laying down position.

Rig: A term for an ambulance.

RMA: *Refused Medical Attention.*

RMA AMA: *Refused Medical Attention Against Medical Advice;* when a patient refuses despite your strongly urging them to go to the hospital.

RMA by Action: When a patient refuses medical help by running away from you or attacking you.

Run: A call.

Run Report: The chart you fill out for a call.

SCBA: *Self-Contained Breathing Apparatus;* the air system worn by firefighters.

Shock: To deliver an electric current to reverse irregular heart rhythms. Also refers to a life threatening condition.

SOB: *Shortness of breath.*

Spike Up: To use heroin intravenously.

Stair Chair: A carrying device that is a collapsible chair, which enables the rescuer to carry a patient down stairs in the seated position.

TB: *Tuberculosis.*

TIA: *Transient Ischemic Attack,* a mini-stroke.

Tour Chief: The immediate supervisor for most ambulance personnel.

Triage Nurse: Nurse in the ER who handles judging the order of who gets treated first based on severity of illness/injury, or degree of smell.

Trauma Alert: Alerts the ER that a serious injury is coming in.

Trauma Center: A hospital that is specialized in treating serious injuries.

Trauma Strip: To cut someone's clothes off for the purpose of assessing injuries or creating an inconvenience to the patient who is obviously bullshitting you.

Trauma Team: A special team of doctors and nurses that handles the more serious injury calls.

Tube a Patient: To place a tube down a patient's airway to facilitate oxygen delivery to the lungs.

Turn-Out Gear: The protective equipment a firefighter wears.

Vital Signs: The patient's pulse, blood pressure, respiratory rate, temperature, etc.

Vollie: A member of a volunteer department.

White Coats: Fire chiefs.

White Shirts: Tour chiefs.

WNL: *Within Normal Limits*; the patient's vital signs are in the normal range for him or her.

A Worker: A confirmed fire. *Proper use:* "They've got a *worker* down on Grand Street."

The following are some other terms used by EMTs on the street. No harm is intended to any particular group of person.

ABC: For the street EMT it means *Ambulate Before Carrying*, another very important assessment tool: check to see if they can walk before you throw your back out carrying them.

Ambulance Dance: The frantic waving of the arms that bystanders believe will actually make you hurry up. The more frantic the waving, the more likely that the call is absolute bullshit. The more frantic, stupid looking dancing is sometimes called the **Ambulance Macarena**. Here's how you judge what's inside: If they continue to dance when you pull up, it's probably not that serious; when they wave their arm once and hightail it inside, worry. (a.k.a. *The Hurry Up Hula*.)

ART: Another important assessment tool; *Assuming Room Temperature*, what the body does when it dies.

The Big One: This is the great call too many people sit around waiting for. Usually, the more you hope for it, the less likely it will come.

Big Red: The fire department.

Big Red House Markers: Fire department first responders. *Proper use:* "Unit 5 will be on scene with the Big Red House Marker."

Bi-Monthly Insult: The paycheck.

Blue Testers: Police officers who run into a potentially hazardous scene. If they come out alive, then you have nothing to worry about, if they turn blue, run the other way. (a.k.a *Cop-o-meters*.)

BLS: *Basic Lifting Service.*

Bompee: An undesirable person.

Buffa Job: to respond to someone else's call, whether it is to handle the call yourself, or just to watch.

Bug Zapper: The defibrillator.

Can Opener: A large, six-cell flashlight that some people carry, not for light, but for times of trouble. "Open a Can of Ass-Whup!" Also known as *The Answer* (to a violent patient).

Cellitis: The unexplainable syndrome that effects most prisoners when they are locked up and face overwhelming evidence of their guilt. Usually characterized by mysterious body aches or fake seizures, or any other type of miscellaneous abnormalities.

Clusterfuck or Charlie Foxtrot: A scene that becomes very chaotic because everyone is doing their own thing.

Code Blue: In the field: signifies that members of the media are on the scene and that everyone should try their hardest to strike a pose that would get their picture in the paper or on the news.

Code Brown: A warning that feces are present on the patient or in the scene.

Concrete Poisoning: What a suicidal jumper dies from. (a.k.a. Anaphylaxis to concrete); the allergic reaction to concrete.

CTD: *Circling the Drain*, a patient whose condition is getting rapidly worse.

Doc in a Box: The medical control doctor who communicates with paramedics on the radio.

DRT: *Dead Right There.*

Doing the Nasty: Cleaning up your ambulance after a messy call.

The Dope Fairy: A being like Santa Claus; we've heard about him, never seen him. He visits people, and without them knowing it, sprinkles them with his magic dope dust. These are fine upstanding citizens who swear they don't do drugs, yet we find them unconscious from an overdose. It *must* be the Dope Fairy.

Drop Test: A sure-fire way to tell if someone is faking being unconscious. Take their arm and drop it on their face. If it doesn't hit them square in the nose, they're not unconscious. If it does hit them in the nose, they're probably unconscious. Drop it again to make sure, or for a laugh.

Duck: A firefighter.

EMS: Earn Money Sleeping.

EMT: Every Menial Task.

Flipper: someone having a seizure.

FNG: Fucking new guy.

FOS: Full of Shit; used primarily by the nurses in the ER to describe many of the frequent visitors: "Uh-oh, here comes FOS again."

Frequent Flyer: Someone who is constantly calling for the ambulance, either for legitimate or BS reasons.

Funkdify: When a dirty patient dirties the back of your truck. The process of cleaning this mess is called *defunkdification.*

Green Gas and Salt Water: Miracle treatment: Oxygen and an IV. No matter what the patient's problem is, we always seem to give them these two things.

HHS: Hysterical Hispanic Syndrome; the predictable reaction by most older Hispanic women, characterized by blowing the situation out of proportion, frantic flailing of the arms, and hyperventilation.

Hitchhiker: A cockroach or other bug that makes a home inside of your ear.

Ho Hunt: The great EMS past time of driving through the streets late at night picking out the hookers.

HVLT: High Velocity Lead Treatment; a gunshot.

Litmus Test: Narcan. If it wakes the patient up, then despite his denials, the chances are very good he was taking heroin because Narcan doesn't work on anything else we know of yet.

Lizard: A really old person.

Lizard-slinging: Interfacility transportation services for really old people.

LOLIND: Little Old Lady in No Distress; an old lady that calls the ambulance with nothing really wrong with her; she's just looking for company.

Mother's Day: The day in the first week of the month when welfare mothers get their checks. This signals the beginning of a busy weekend of assaults, overdoses, and general all around anarchy and mayhem.

NMS: New Mother Syndrome; characterized by freaking out over the slightest things, like the baby crying.

Nut Truck: a mobile crisis team.

Olfactory Emergency: A condition in which the patient's stench is unbearably nasty.

Paramagicians: Paramedics; may also be **paragods** depending upon the size of their ego.

Positive "O" Sign: One way to tell if someone is dead is by the expression on their face that looks like they are saying "O." This changes, however, to the **Positive "Q" Sign** when the patient's tongue is hanging out.

Prudential Syndrome: The group of symptoms, including neck, back, and head pain that follows minor MVAs. Usually the result of your insurance swelling. (a.k.a. *Allstate-itis*)

Prodigy: A person who does stupid things, like riding their bicycle down the middle of the road dressed in black at midnight and wondering why they got hit by a bus.

Pumpkin: A person who has overdosed on heroin. When they overdose, they go to sleep and begin to snore like a baby. So you pat them on the head and say, "Night, night pumpkin." **Narcan** is also known as the **Anti-Pumpkin Juice**.

The "Q" Word: *Quiet.* This is the most dreaded of all words to an EMT on duty. To utter it almost guarantees that your day will be anything but.

Skell: Can mean any undesirable person but is usually reserved for fellow coworkers.

Skate: An EMT who wastes as much time as possible in order to avoid more work.

Skid: An undesirable person.

Slim Shady or Slim Pickens: A very large patient.

Smoke: A crack user.

Smurfing: When the patient in respiratory distress begins to turn blue.

SOB: Considering what section it's in, what do you think it means?

Spooge: Disgusting body fluids that spew forth from a patient.

Squirrel: A firefighter or EMT who responds to other people's calls.

Stealth Taxi: When you turn off all the lights and sirens, honk the horn, and have the patient walk to the ambulance.

TIA: A brain fart, when you forget what you were going to say.

TMI: Too Much Information; when the patient, or anyone for that matter, let's you know more than you needed, or wanted, to know.

Turf Granny Day: The Friday that precedes a very nice or long weekend when home health aids call the ambulance for made up emergencies so they can have the weekend off while grandma is in the hospital.

"Two Dude" Syndrome: The only explanation possible when you find the junkie or hooker on the corner who just got the crap beaten out of him or her and they swear they don't know what happened. "You see, he was standing on the corner, not doing nothing, when these two dudes that I never seen before came up and jumped him for no reason at all."

Urine Express: The elevator in a housing project high-rise.

Whacker: Someone who takes the position of EMT way too seriously.

Wig Out: When a patient (or co-worker) goes crazy.

Whiz Quiz: A urine test administered when you get into an accident with the ambulance.

WNL: *We Never Looked.*

Wrinkle Ranch: A nursing home. (a.k.a. *Geriatric Park.*)